Advance Praise for *Taking Charge*

You don't have to feel helpless any more! *Taking Charge* enables you to understand and embrace your vital role in helping prevent common medical complications in your elderly loved one.

> WENDY S. HARPHAM, MD, FACP, author of *Happiness in a Storm:*
> *Facing Illness and Embracing Life as a Healthy Survivor*

Taking Charge will help caregivers learn about illnesses that commonly affect the elderly, about medicines often prescribed for the elderly, and about common and sometimes fatal adverse reactions to drugs. This new book focuses on helping caregivers initiate preventive measures to ensure longer, healthier lives for their loved ones.

> JOEL SHUSTER, PharmD, BCPP, Clinical Professor of Pharmacy
> Temple University School of Pharmacy, Philadelphia, PA, USA
> and Trustee Institute for Safe Medication Practices.

This book eloquently captures the sense of helplessness felt by family caregivers and their loved ones when conditions that commonly affect the elderly result in a downward spiral. Jeanne Hannah describes her experience and the lessons she wants to share with you so that you can protect your loved one by helping her doctors detect, resolve, and prevent these conditions.

> RONALD F. PFEIFFER, MD, Professor and Vice Chair of the Department
> of Neurology at the University of Tennessee (Memphis). Co-editor
> (with Manuchair Ebadi) of the book "*Parkinson's Disease*," published by
> CRC Press in 2005, and awarded first prize in the neurology category in
> the 2005 British Medical Association's Medical Book Competition.

Inappropriate use of psychiatric drugs can have a devastating impact on our elderly. Yet each year, countless seniors are given these drugs to treat delirium misdiagnosed as psychosis or dementia, rather than treating the underlying cause of an elder patient's illness, often something as common and treatable as a urinary tract infection. *Taking Charge* is nothing short of a manual on how to get the best medical care for your loved one.

> LEE SPILLER, Executive Director, Citizens Commission
> on Human Rights of Texas

OLD MISSION PRESS
WEBSITE:
http://goodmedicalcare.com
READ & PRINT APPENDICES

Taking Charge

Taking Charge

Good Medical Care for the Elderly and How to Get It

Jeanne M. Hannah

Attorney, Trial Lawyer, and Caregiver

and

Joseph H. Friedman, M.D.

Professor, Department of Clinical Neurosciences
Brown University School of Medicine

Old Mission Press

Old Mission, Michigan

FIRST EDITION

Publisher Cataloging-in-Publication Data
Hannah, Jeanne M., 1941–
Taking charge : good medical care for the elderly and how to get it / Jeanne M. Hannah with a chapter by Joseph H. Friedman. 1st edition.
p. cm.
Includes endnotes (p.219) and index.
ISBN 0–9779837–0–6
ISBN 13 978–0–97–798370–4

1. Aging—Caregivers manual—United States. 2. Aging—Health—United States. 3. Aging Medication safe practices—United States. 4. Aging—Preventive care—United States. 5. Aging—Nutrition—United States. I. Friedman, Joseph H. Title.
HQ1063.6.H36 2006
362.6—dc22   2006904703

This book is available at special discounts when purchased in bulk for premiums and sales promotions and well as for fundraising or educational use. Special editions or book excerpts can also be created to specification. For details contact the publisher at the address below:

Old Mission Press
P.O. Box 9
Old Mission, Michigan 49673

Email: jeannemhannah@pentel.net

Printed in the United States on recycled paper.

First printing June 2006

10 9 8 7 6 5 4 3 2 1

This book is dedicated to my mother,

ALICE MARIE SCHMITTGEN

Contents

Contents

NOTICE

This book is not intended as a medical manual. Rather, it is intended as a reference volume and the information included is given to help you make informed decisions about your health and the health of your loved ones. This volume is not intended to be a substitute for any care, treatment, diagnosis or supervision that may be prescribed by a physician. If you think that you or someone for whom you care has a medical problem, you are urged to seek competent professional medical advice.

Wherever possible, the authors have included only the name of generic medications, however, from time to time brand names are given as an example. The appropriateness of any medication, other product, or treatment should be decided by you or your loved one in consultation with a physician.

Internet addresses (URLs), mailing addresses and telephone numbers provided in this book were accurate and functional at the time this book went to press.

Acknowledgments

As I labored to discover the cause of Mom's death and then to share this story with others whose loved ones might be in danger, I found extraordinary contributors whose efforts inspired me to dig deeper and to advocate more wisely, whose knowledge and expertise were invaluable, whose dedication to the health and well-being of the elderly was awe-inspiring, and whose assistance and encouragement were willingly and freely given. I express gratitude and appreciation to the following individuals. Their insight informed my opinions and made this book possible:

Wendy S. Harpham, M.D., author of *Happiness in a Storm: Facing Life and Embracing Happiness as a Healthy Survivor*; *Diagnosis Cancer: Your Guide Through the First Few Months*; and others, inspired me with her unflagging advocacy as a physician-educator and with her courage. Dr. Harpham's enthusiastic and caring mentorship was invaluable as I sought to bring what I learned to publication. Dr. Harpham read two of the later manuscripts, made thoughtful suggestions about making the material reader-friendly, and helped me to clarify the message about the importance of communication with doctors and other medical caregivers. Without her generous assistance, this book would never have come into fruition.

Dr. John E. Morley, the Director of the Division of Geriatric Medicine and the Dammert Professor of Gerontology at Saint Louis University Medical School, urged me to write this book, for he believes that families and caregivers really need the information provided here. He encouraged me to help families learn to communicate with the physicians who provide care to the elderly and helped me understand the complicated issues of dehydration and malnutrition.

Joseph H. Friedman, M.D., Professor of Clinical Neurosciences at Brown University, has generously contributed his medical expertise as co-author of this book. Dr. Friedman is known for his responsible use of psychotropic medications in Parkinson's disease patients, and his ability to see the interrelationships and complexities of the medical issues that are at the core of this book has provided a clarity of focus for the reader.

Mark H. Beers, M.D., Editor-in-Chief of The Merck Manual and The Merck Manual of Geriatrics and Executive Director of Geriatrics and Clinical Literature at Merck & Co., Inc., encouraged me and provided me with valuable insights into how medications may be used responsibly in the elderly. His knowledge and expertise guided my efforts, and his advocacy inspired me.

Joel Shuster, PharmD, BCPP, Professor of Clinical Pharmacy, Temple University School of Pharmacy, Philadelphia, Pennsylvania, sent me references, answered my questions about medications, side effects and medication errors, reviewed the chapters on dehydration and medication errors and encouraged me every step of the way.

John O. Zachman, M.D., a tireless and dedicated internist practicing in Traverse City, Michigan, has been my personal physician for many years. John agreed to become Mom's attending physician at my request so that we could move her to Traverse City. Neither of us knew that we were getting such a desperately ill patient. John's attendance at Mom's bedside was unwavering. He communicated with us in a caring and sensitive manner. Most of all, John was attentive to end-of-life issues, in particular the management of pain, for which we are grateful indeed.

Sharon Olson, Ph.D., R.N., C.S., established the Palliative Care Center on the Old Mission Peninsula near Traverse City, Michigan. A gerontologist, nurse practitioner, and gentle harpist with healing hands and heart, Sharon helped me understand palliative care and hospice care through her fine example and gave me the courage to choose hospice care for Mom. She read an early manuscript and offered gentle and apt suggestions.

My editor, Rebecca Chown, through her endearing enthusiasm and cheerful competence, made revisions the easiest part of this writing process. Without her help and expertise, this book would not exist.

Several other people are deserving of gratitude: my sisters Elizabeth Hickey and Jill Eurick who helped as caregivers during Mom's last illness; Mary Kay McDuffie, Don Orr, Mary Lynn Teter, and Verley Ward, friends who read the first and later drafts, and Kathleen Cole and Lija Ditmar, friends who offered encouragement and suggestions, particularly in the latter stages of research and writing.

Taking Charge

Introduction

In 2000, I became a family caregiver for a very short period in time—65 days, to be exact. In the fall of 2000, my bright, active, and independent 84-year-old mother became ill with a urinary tract infection (UTI). This was correctly diagnosed at the emergency room of a local hospital. What was not diagnosed was the delirium that was caused by this infection, even though disease-induced delirium is common in the elderly. At the time her illness began, Mom lived in her own home with my youngest sister, Jill. Despite the best efforts and intentions of Jill, our other sister Betsy, and myself, Mom died only 65 days later. This book is written with the hope that you, a family caregiver, or you—a "baby-boomer" whose health may impacted by common and preventable conditions, will avoid the tragic result that occurred with my mother. Knowledge is power. If you can learn the simple preventative measures that can prevent medical and medication errors for yourself or a loved one, then my mission will be complete.

The symptoms of Mom's delirium—visual and auditory delusions—led to a psychiatric hospitalization. There, drugs that are dangerous to the elderly—antipsychotic drugs that interacted with her medications for her Parkinson's disease and blocked their healthy effect—led to serious complications. The complications caused by the drug-drug and drug-disease interactions were misinterpreted by her doctors and nurses. They were understood to be a worsening of her Parkinson's disease, and were not interpreted as medication errors or medication interactions. She declined rapidly. Her body systems failed. Since none of the medications she normally took and none of the medications that the facility prescribed for her to "cure" the symptoms that were observed were eliminated or reduced, her kidneys could not fully eliminate the many drugs going into her body. She died, then, because she was "poisoned." The primary cause of death listed by the pathologist on the autopsy report was "toxic encephalopathy"— brain death—death caused by her brain being overwhelmed by toxic substances so that it could not enable her normal life processes to continue.

I subsequently learned that Mom died because of several developing complications that commonly affect the elderly, whether they live in their own home, a caregiver's home, or a long-term care facility. I learned that these complications are predictable, often caused by a medical or medication error, recognizable, treatable, and preventable. I learned that early detection is key to successful treatment, and prevention is the goal caregivers must strive for. I also learned that a family caregiver can be and must be the first line of defense for her elderly loved one.

My mother's last days were horrible, and her death was very traumatic for me, primarily because I felt so responsible. After all, I'd made the choices—or participated with my sisters in making choices—that had led to her death. I set about to figure out exactly why she had died. After all, she'd only had a minor UTI. What I learned is that when an elderly person becomes ill, very often complications of the illness itself, or complications arising from a treatment or a medication, can cause something like a domino effect. There are so many ways in which one problem can quickly create another and another.

I've since been impelled to share with other caregivers what I've learned about six common and often fatal conditions that affect the elderly so that other family caregivers can avoid the tragedy that befell our mother and our family. My research revealed to me that Mom's death was caused by a progression of problems that could easily have been prevented: (1) delirium, (2) medication errors, (3) adverse drug reactions, (4) dehydration, and (5) malnutrition. These five complications commonly cause death in the elderly. Falls causing injuries are a sixth common cause of death in the elderly, and all six are preventable! These six potentially fatal medical problems are thoroughly presented in this book.

My mother's urinary tract infection was diagnosed in the emergency room of a hospital in the city where she lived in mid-Michigan, a three-hour drive from my home. Subsequently, she was confined and treated in a local nursing facility, spending two weeks in a psychiatric unit, two weeks in a medical, and almost three weeks in a "rehabilitative care" unit. Thus her care was provided by four different medical teams—all doctors and nurses who did not know her—and there was no continuity of care. I had no way of knowing then how vital continuity of care was in properly assessing and diagnosing Mom's emerging symptoms and how, as a result, lack of diagnosis and appropriate medical care caused serious conditions to escalate and overwhelm her body.

My sisters visited Mom every day. I talked with her on the telephone every day, but I saw her much less frequently. It soon became apparent that

Mom was not improving and was, in fact, getting much worse. I asked the staff about many of her symptoms showing her decline. But when I questioned the nurses about them, I was told repeatedly that these changes were "to be expected," that Mom was "debilitated," and that there was "nothing that could be done."

Looking back, it is fair to say that Mom was treated as many elderly persons are today: she was written off. There was a pervasive attitude among the caregivers I encountered in the long-term care facility that the patients were old and were going to die anyway, that caring for them—changing diapers, hand-feeding—was something that the workers did, not because they liked to do it, wanted to do it, or were even particularly good at it, but because they needed the minimum wages that are paid for these unpleasant jobs.

I decided to transfer Mom to a nursing facility near my home so that I could have more direct access to her and help with her care. I did not realize how critically ill Mom was on the morning I picked her up to take her to Traverse City, nor did the doctors or nurses tell me. The nursing facility had done lab tests that morning. Had they reviewed them, or had they even provided me with copies of them, perhaps things would have worked out differently. Those lab tests, which I found in Mom's medical records after her death, revealed that she was so critically dehydrated that she should have been transported immediately to a hospital.

Why weren't my sisters and I more forceful or more adept at getting proper medical treatment for Mom? At the time she was admitted to the nursing home, my sisters and I thought it best to leave her care to the staff. We were intimidated because we had no particular knowledge of geriatric medical matters and we assumed the staff had critical knowledge we did not possess. We did not realize that these doctors and nurses, like most doctors and nurses, had no training at all in geriatrics, as Dr. Friedman explains in Chapter One. Sadly, we did not appreciate the importance of our intimate knowledge of Mom's usual mental acuity and her normal physical abilities and limitations. Nor did we realize how our assessment of changes in Mom's mental and physical condition, if communicated to her medical caregivers, could have led to diagnosis and treatment of critical, emerging, fatal conditions. In particular, we did not realize that our communications of changes in her status to nurses were minimized because the nurses' assessments were based only on what they saw, and were not seen in perspective with observations made a few weeks earlier when she was in the care of a different team.

What I now know could have saved my mom's life and may save the life of your loved one.[1] I now know that the primary caregiver is the person most likely to know when a loved one needs medical attention. I thought Mom's doctors and nurses were monitoring her care. I was shocked when my research revealed that a person living in a nursing home may see a physician *once a month for five to 15 minutes!* That same person may have some attention daily from a nurse, either an LPN or an RN, but usually LPNs and RNs spend *less than one hour per day* per resident. Much of that time is spent doing indirect care such as writing nursing notes or preparing medications for distribution. Residents of nursing homes do get about two hours of care per day from a competency evaluated nurse assistant (CENA), but CENAs are typically responsible for the care of 12 to 14 residents in an 8-hour shift and are not trained in medicine. They are usually entry-level employees with minimal training and experience. They not only lack the education and training to detect signs of medical complications, they haven't the time to look for them.

The elderly patient, if competent, is in the best position to detect that something is wrong, that something has changed in her condition. If she is unable to communicate effectively or to understand and appreciate changes in her condition—if, for example, she is suffering from dementia—then a family caregiver who undoubtedly spends more time with her than her medical caregivers is the best person to detect these changes, even without special training. A family caregiver who sees something different about the way a loved one is functioning physically or mentally can and should tell a primary care physician and follow up with an appointment.

While my sisters and I were intimidated by our lack of medical expertise and by what we thought to be the complexities of Mom's medical treatment, I have since learned that there are tools and knowledge that family members can use to help keep their elderly loved ones healthy and safe. After a great deal of research, I have been able to understand how ordinary—how common, in fact—Mom's medical problems were and how capable we might have been in helping her caregivers assess changes in her condition. I have come to appreciate the critical role a family caregiver can play in early diagnosis of medical conditions and, more importantly, in

---

[1] Recognizing that the person for whom you are a caregiver may be your parent, grandparent, or spouse, and sometimes an adult child, the term "loved one" is used consistently. To avoid continuous awkwardness, the pronouns "she," "her," and "hers" will be used rather than constructions like "him or her." Indeed, since most family caregivers are themselves 60 or older, the information in this book will apply to their own healthcare as well.

the prevention of these medical conditions. In my case, what I did not know hurt my mom and resulted in her death from terrible and preventable conditions.

This book is my gift to you and your loved one: the easy lessons I learned too late, the lessons that would have saved my dear mother, and the lessons that could save your loved one. I want you and your loved one to be spared the suffering and death my mom endured and the loss our family experienced as a result.

If you are caring for an elderly loved one, or if you are 65 years old or older, *Taking Charge: Good Medical Care for the Elderly and How to Get It* will give you the information and tools you need to form an effective alliance with physicians and caregivers. Let me emphasize that medical training is not required for this task.

Let me also reassure you that my goal in this book is not to convince you that nursing homes are horrible dungeons that the elderly must avoid at all costs. Many elderly persons experience healing, productive stays in a nursing facility when recovering from surgery, stroke, or other illnesses requiring hospitalization, rehabilitation, and recuperation. However, nursing homes do have, in general, some serious shortcomings—notably a lack of adequate staffing, which you will read about in Chapter Eight. To protect your loved one from the possibility that understaffing may result in harm, you need to know when to sound the alert that will bring assistance from physicians and nurses and how to work with them to prevent your loved one from falling victim to common preventable medical complications. Your willingness and ability to enter into an alliance with the physicians and the nurses overseeing your loved one's care will make you a valuable asset to her medical caregivers.

I believe you will find the information presented in this book, if frightening at first, enlightening and empowering over the long haul. Each chapter is organized to help you to recognize the symptoms of these common conditions and to understand why your loved one is at risk for them. Armed with this vital information, you will be able to describe changes in your loved one's status to her physician so that early diagnosis and treatment can prevent her downward spiral and early death. Most important of all, prevention is key to your loved one's health. The information provided here will help you minimize the risks and prevent the onset of common complications that can pose a significant threat to your loved one's health and life. My goal is to give you the tools you need and to encourage you to have the confidence needed to communicate effectively with your loved one's medical caregivers.

Endnotes containing the medical journal articles I relied on are found at the back of the book so that you may determine the source of statistics and other technical information. If you want more detailed information, your local librarian will be able to order any of these articles for you. Many of the sources upon which I relied are available on the Internet. I've provided the URLs for these. I found some articles to be so valuable and so universally relevant that I placed references to them in Appendix P as "Recommended Readings." You will find other appendices helpful as well. All appendices are available without charge on the Internet where they may be read onine or printed out. The primary reasons why these materials are available on the Internet is that they are more useful to you as 8- by 10-inch pages that you can three-hole punch and keep in a binder as part of your loved one's "care-giver's record," and also there are many hyperlinks in the appendices which will make it easier for you to access the tools, the articles, and the associations to which you will be referred.

As a lawyer, I have always told my clients, "Knowledge is power. What you don't know can hurt you." Use this knowledge to prevent harm to your loved one.

March 1, 2006
Old Mission, Michigan

CHAPTER ONE

Why the Elderly Can't Get Good Medical Care

BY JOSEPH H. FRIEDMAN, M.D.

Doctors and Nurses Have Little or No Training in Geriatrics

As a physician and educator, (I teach at Brown University Medical School), I know better than most that it is no longer possible for families and caregivers to depend upon doctors and nurses to protect their elderly loved ones. Instead, families and caregivers themselves must work to maintain the elderly patient's good health. The problem? Doctors and nurses caring for the elderly have little or no training in geriatrics. The pharmacists who fill their prescriptions and who may recommend over-the-counter drugs to them likewise have little or no training in geriatrics.

For this reason, it is critical to the daily health and well-being of the elderly that their families and caregivers learn about the common diseases and conditions that are potentially fatal to them. Family caregivers must learn to communicate to doctors and nurses any changes in a patient's condition they see, for such changes signal what could become a serious crisis. They must also learn to assess what makes a loved one at risk for deadly conditions and how to reduce these risks as a preventative measure. They should strive for continuity of care so that her doctors and nurses will be more likely to perceive important status changes as a warning sign that the patient is experiencing a potentially deadly complication.

Because of their lack of knowledge, physicians, nurses, and other healthcare providers often fail to recognize the potential for drug interactions, symptoms of adverse drug reactions, or new disease processes and instead misunderstand these to be part of the natural aging process. As a result, experts say that millions of older Americans face greater risks of potentially fatal complications such as these:

- getting the wrong diagnosis
- having a potentially fatal condition or disease go undiagnosed
- having the wrong medication prescribed for them
- not getting a proper and necessary medication prescribed for them
- being harmed by innocent misuse of prescription drugs and/or over-the-counter drugs
- having a drug-drug, drug-food, or drug-disease interaction that will be fatal if it goes undetected

These are only some of the things that can go wrong. In February 2002, the Alliance for Aging Research released a report documenting the grave shortage of trained healthcare workers called "Medical Never-Never Land: 10 Reasons Why America Is Not Ready for the Coming Age Boom."[1] The report describes the magnitude of the crisis in healthcare for the elderly and also makes clear the lack of a reasonable prospect for a solution in the near future. As a result, your loved one may be at risk unless you are able and willing to learn about the diseases and conditions that pose the most serious threats and also are able and willing to be a member of her caregiving team.

If you wish to know why doctors, nurses, and other medical caregivers lack critical training in geriatrics, you can find a short summary of the Alliance for Aging Research report in the endnotes for this chapter. You can also read the entire report on the Internet or download it to your computer.[2] What you, as a family caregiver, must know is how much at risk your loved one is and how to protect her from potentially fatal complications. In fact, if you are a Baby Boomer yourself, as most caregivers are, what you learn in this book about common diseases and conditions affecting the elderly will help you to protect your own health!

I also hope this book will aid in your self-confidence: you are the individual most capable of observing and detecting the changes, even subtle changes, that tell you there is something very wrong with your loved one.

Finally, this book is intended to help you learn how to communicate your observations to doctors and nurses so that your loved one is properly diagnosed and treated. If you don't, the possibilities are great that your elderly loved one will be marginalized, or essentially "written off." This occurs far too often, particularly in the institutional setting.

How the Elderly Differ from the Population at Large

Because many, if not most, healthcare professionals are not trained in geriatrics, they often fail to recognize the health needs of older adults. Appropriate care for the elderly depends upon focusing on the unique way in which the elderly differ from younger patients, for a change in condition can signal a deadly disease or a drug interaction that, if not addressed, can prove fatal.

Specifically, the elderly often have symptoms that differ from those of younger persons with the same illness. For example, an older person who has a heart attack may not experience crushing chest pain but only dizziness and confusion. Or, an individual with hypothyroidism may appear to be suffering from dementia. Delirium, a sign of a life-threatening disease or condition that urgently needs treatment, is often mistaken by physicians and nurses as dementia. The result is that the elderly patient may not be diagnosed properly and treated appropriately, and death may result.

Elderly patients also face potentially hazardous interactions from drugs prescribed by different practitioners. Some doctors do not know that older people metabolize certain drugs differently from younger people, thus exposing elderly patients to inappropriate dosages that can cause harm and sometimes death.

The difficulties in managing and treating the elderly are made far more complex by the fact that the body's response to medications is markedly different among the various age groups within that group we refer to as "the elderly." You should look at your elderly loved one like this: age 65-75 is "young old," 75-85 is "older old," and 85 and older is "oldest old." When treating these patients with medications, the drugs must be carefully tailored, both in choice and dosage, to each individual, taking into consideration her health history, her known diseases, and also her existing drug regimen to avoid the medication errors and adverse drug reactions that will be discussed in detail in later chapters. These drugs should also be re-evaluated if the patient's kidneys begin to fail, as often occurs in the elderly either as a normal effect of aging or as the result of an emerging condition such as dehydration, so that dosages may be tapered or eliminated to protect the patient from toxicity and death.

Your Loved One Needn't Always See a Geriatrician

Most elderly are cared for by general internists and family physicians. Not every patient needs to be seen by a geriatrician, a specialist in aging-related health issues and gerontology. Whether a geriatrician is needed is based more on a patient's particular healthcare needs than on her chronological age. Two individuals both aged 65 may have very different degrees of disability or illness; one may have no problems at all while the other may have serious health concerns. Geriatricians frequently provide the primary care for older adults who have complicated medical and social problems. But for most elderly patients, an occasional consultation with a geriatrician who can then advise the primary care physician is sufficient.

If a patient becomes critically ill, a primary care physician may call in other specialists to consult. She may involve a geriatrician, whose major goal would be to coordinate the work of specialists and other healthcare providers such as social workers, nurses, and home health aides. The medical caregiving team may include, with or without a geriatrician, any or all of the following professionals:

- Nurse
- Social worker
- Nutritionist
- Physical therapist
- Occupational therapist
- Consultant pharmacist
- Geropsychiatrist

The members of this team look at each patient holistically. The team considers the patient's medical history and present health condition. The team also looks for the effects of past illnesses as well as "geriatric syndromes"—health problems frequently found in the frail elderly such as incontinence, frequent falls, depression, memory problems, and the side effects caused by multiple medications. The team's purpose is to detect, treat, and prevent the geriatric syndromes that are a direct threat to the elderly patient's ability to live independently. Again, while not all health professionals need to be certified in geriatric care and not every elderly person needs a geriatrician, a geriatrician should be consulted when:

- Your loved one's condition causes considerable impairment and frailty. For example, she may be over the age of 75 and coping with

a number of diseases and disabilities, including cognitive problems
such as dementia
* Use of numerous prescription drugs makes it unclear which drugs
are appropriate and which may be causing additional problems
* Family members and friends are feeling considerable stress and
strain as caregivers

Caregivers—an Essential Part of the Caregiving Team

As a family caregiver, you can be a valuable and effective member of the
caregiving team. As you will read often in this book, the likelihood is great
that you are the person who spends the most time with your elderly loved
one and that you are the one in the best position to observe changes in her
condition that indicate something is very wrong—that she's suffering from
a disease process or condition that her physician needs to address right
away.

Let me give you an example: much of what happened to Jeanne's
mother resonates with experiences my patients have had, one of which I
will describe because it illustrates a successful outcome of a determined
daughter's intervention, a good resolution, quite different than Jeanne's.
Mrs. Smith, like Jeanne's mother, had Parkinson's disease. It was so severe
that her elderly husband and married-with-children daughter couldn't care
for her adequately and she was admitted to a long-term care facility.

A month later the daughter called me. "Mom's doing terribly," she said.
"When she went into the nursing home she could walk with a cane part of
the day, feed herself all three meals, walk with a walker to the dining room
all the time, and always assist in her care. Now she can't walk anytime, or
feed herself. She can't do a thing, and I'm sure they screwed up her medication by giving her sustained release instead of immediate release medicine for her Parkinson's disease."

I assured her that such a change, while not endorsed by me, would not
have made such a difference and that I would investigate. I telephoned the
nursing home and had the charge nurse read the names, doses, and sched-
ules of all the medications. I learned that a new medication had been
started to treat the patient's chronic complaint of nausea. This medicine,
unfortunately, causes PD patients to get stiffer and slower, a fact not well
known to most doctors or nurses. I had the medicine stopped and, over the
next few weeks, the patient's mobility returned to its previous level.

What struck me was partly the mistake of prescribing the drug in the first place, but mostly I was struck by the lack of recognition that something bad had happened to the patient. The nausea had improved and no side effects were observed. The nursing staff interpreted this as a success. The worsened motor function was interpreted as disease progression, the natural course of Mrs. Smith's Parkinson's disease. After all, that's why she came into the nursing home in the first place. What the staff failed to recognize was that the parkinsonism Mrs. Smith was exhibiting—increased tremor, stiffness, lack of mobility—was an adverse drug reaction. Here was an obvious, inadvertent, and correctable problem that occurred at a good nursing home with what passes for adequate staffing these days.

Fortunately, because of a vigilant advocate, a caring staff, and a doctor who had experience with the type of adverse drug reaction this patient suffered and who is committed to being available to his patients and their families, Mrs. Smith is still walking and feeding herself. But how often, I asked myself, is this happening where the family believes the staff's reassurances that this sudden worsening represents the disease's ceaseless progression? When family members hear comments like "It's so sad; we see this all the time. There's nothing you can do," most take them at face value.

It's important that you tell your loved one's doctor what you see—changes that may indicate a serious problem. Don't diagnose the problem yourself, because you may hinder the way her doctor analyzes the situation. Just make a list of all symptoms you observe and concerns you have and share them with the doctor either by telephone, telefax, or in person. Doctors rely upon checklists to help them assess and rule out the possible causes of such problems. They begin by considering the most common problems, and often find the answer they are looking at without having to complete an entire battery of tests. Then treatment of the emerging condition can begin promptly and often disaster can be averted. So if you learn more about the conditions Jeanne will address in this book, you will learn what to look for, how to communicate what you see to her doctors and nurses, and how to prevent these conditions from occuring so that your elderly loved one's life is longer, richer, safer, and more independent.

Conclusion

While I am no expert on nursing homes, I do know something about them. My grandmother suffered from Parkinson's disease when I was a child, before the development of L-Dopa, the main drug used for treating it. I clearly recall the nursing home she was in and the emotional problems her illness caused for the family. Likewise, I have a lot of patients who visit from nursing homes. I like to think I am observant, and I have a fair amount of common sense. As Yogi Berra reportedly said, "You can see a lot just by looking."

One reason Jeanne's mother was seen so little in the nursing home was that doctor payments are very low. My veterinarian receives more money for a routine evaluation of my healthy cat than I get for seeing people with Parkinson's disease, and she's not overpaid! For a time I "moonlighted" doing EMGs, a neurological test for diagnosing pinched nerves. I was paid approximately eight times, sometime ten times, as much as I would have been paid to spend an hour with a new PD patient. Seeing a patient with Alzheimer's disease and talking with her family about her myriad problems is getting to be a money-losing proposition. This translates into reduced time for interactions with the patient, reduced knowledge about the patient, reduced time to gather information from the nurses, reduced time to hear from the family, and less time or no time to actually talk with the family.

As Jeanne articulately explains in later chapters, the lack of contact between physicians, the patient, and family caregivers is frustrating, but it is also frustrating for the doctor. Between the frustration and the low reimbursements, it's no wonder that geriatrics is so under-subscribed.

What this means for you is that while you should try to seek out a geriatrician to care for your elderly loved one, you may not find one, even at a good nursing home. Even if you do find one who is good, you will still need to function as a patient advocate and inform the staff when you see worrisome changes that they don't. You may need, hopefully rarely, to go over the staff's head to the physician directly to communicate a concern. You can send a note or fax and/or request a phone call or a discussion. There is an advertising motto that a clothing store in the northeast has used for decades that I think applies in many situations. I invoke it frequently in my clinical research trials, and I think it applies to nursing homes as well: "An informed customer is our best client."

The nursing home, doctor, patient, and family are all on the same side. We all want what's best for the patient, keeping in mind certain resource limitations. The more informed the patient, staff, and family are, the better everyone can work together to improve the patient and staff's quality of life. Everyone does better when the patient does better. A happier patient makes for a happier family, a happier staff, and a better outcome. Being an advocate does not mean being a pain in the neck. In this book Jeanne tells her story in the hope that the reader will be better prepared to avoid similar problems and to better solve them, should they occur.

CHAPTER TWO

Delirium, Dementia, Depression, and Psychosis: The Importance of a Correct Diagnosis

SEPTEMBER 14, 2000

Glen and I were eating dinner when the telephone rang. I answered. It was my sister Jill, calling from the emergency room of a mid-Michigan hospital to say that Mom had been having bizarre and frightening hallucinations all day. Mom thought "they" were coming for her. She kept describing how "they" were outside the house, circling from window to window, and calling to her, "Alice, you have to come with us. It's time for you to go."

Jill said that Mom told her she'd told "them" they'd have to come back later, that she had her bridge club coming soon. However, Jill also learned that Mom had called her bridge group and told them not to come, that she couldn't play cards today.

According to Jill, Mom had a urinary tract infection (UTI). I learned much later that hallucinations are a common symptom of a UTI with a fever in the elderly. The ER physician who diagnosed Mom told Jill that she could take Mom home, but that someone would have to stay with her to watch her.

Jill had just started back to work after a prolonged absence due to a recurrence of breast cancer. She explained that she could not stay home from work to care for Mom.

Betsy, our other sister, was caring for her critically ill husband, Mike, who had recently undergone heart surgery and who was struggling with lung cancer.

Jill said on the phone that the emergency room physician had explained he could admit Mom to a facility related to the hospital. He described it as a place for people with mental problems. He said that if Mom checked herself in, she would be able to discharge herself, but that if she refused to check herself in, he would admit her involuntarily. Then she would not be able to leave if she wanted to.

Jill asked me if I agreed with a voluntary admission to a mental health facility. That was when I made my first mistake. I agreed that Jill should convince Mom to voluntarily admit herself. Now, when I Monday-morning quarterback, I realize that I should have jumped in the car and driven the three and a half hours to Mom's home. I should either have taken care of her there or brought her back to our house until she got better. A urinary tract infection, properly treated, goes away quickly. With one of the new wonder drugs, you can eliminate a UTI in a matter of two days.

Instead, Jill and Betsy drove Mom to Alpine Manor, the behavioral medicine unit of the facility associated with the hospital where the ER was.[1] It was nearly midnight by the time Mom was admitted and the paperwork completed.

A history was taken and a psychiatric evaluation was done. When questions were asked about prior episodes of "confusion" (a benign way of describing delirium often used in medical literature), one of my sisters answered that, yes, Mom had been confused in the past few weeks or months. She really meant that, as is common with the elderly, Mom would hear something or be told something but later, she would need to be told again. Forgetfulness ("confusion") is common in the elderly.

It was established that Mom had no prior history of mental illness and that there was no family history of mental illness. The initial psychiatric evaluation also said that Mom had demonstrated some memory deficits over the past two years. This record said that her hallucinations began two days earlier. Parkinson's disease and the urinary tract infection (UTI) were noted in the history, as well as the prescription of a powerful antibiotic for the UTI.

On September 15, the medical director, a psychiatrist who had never seen Mom before, diagnosed her not with delirium but instead with a psychotic disorder "possibly secondary to urinary tract infection and/or Parkinson's disease." He noted that it was necessary to "rule out" dementia. He prescribed 0.25 mg of an antianxiety medication to treat her extreme paranoid anxiety. An antipsychotic was prescribed on September 17 for her "acute anxiety that was accompanied by bizarre hallucinations."

I did not go down to see Mom the first two weeks she was in Alpine Manor. The visiting hours were from 6:00 p.m. until 7:00 p.m.; it seemed impossible to travel seven hours for a one-hour visiting period. Jill and Betsy were visiting with her daily and there was an 800 number I could call so that I could talk with her every day. Some days, I called her twice. The hope was that the infection would soon go away and she'd feel better and would be able to go home.

Each day that I talked with her, Mom would begin the telephone call with a long list of "news." The problem with the "news" was that it was one story after another of simply horrible things that had happened to a family member. Each time Mom would recount a story about how Michelle had had a bad accident with Mom's car, I'd say, "No, Mom, that was just a bad dream. It didn't happen. Everything is okay, Michelle and the car, too."

Mom would then tell me about Kathy's husband, Brian, a policeman (Kathy was one of Mom's granddaughters). "Did you know that Brian got shot yesterday and died?" Mom would ask.

"No, Mom, that was another bad dream. It really didn't happen," I would reply.

At the time, it was difficult for me to understand why Mom kept having all of these horrible thoughts. It was not until long after her death that I learned that hallucinations and paranoid thoughts are a common symptom of delirium and that many factors endemic to nursing homes contribute to delirium and/or confusion in elderly people. I learned that it is important to give emotional support to delirious patients, to acknowledge their concerns and reassure them that things are all right, rather than to deny their delusions. I also learned that when, as with Mom, delirium is undiagnosed, the result for the frail elderly patient may be imminent death.

Mom's hallucinations continued unabated and, according to the nursing notes that I eventually read, became more severe. Mom had slept during the night, according to the nursing notes, the first few days after her admission. However, between September 17 and 19, Mom slept very little; instead, she wandered the halls. At 6:45 a.m. on September 19, when she was encouraged by an elderly male patient who had befriended her to wave her cane at the monsters she was seeing and her cane struck a staff member, Mom was diagnosed as psychotic. Her medical records simply reflect that she "assaulted" a staff person. The antipsychotic was immediately doubled. There was nothing in her records to indicate that there had been any inquiry into the background of the incident— something that would have established that this was an isolated incident and was not evidence that Mom was dangerous to other people.

It was the beginning of the end. After the "assault," the staff transferred Mom to the intensive care section of the facility and took away her cane, which she used because of her Parkinson's disease. She was not given a walker, nor was Jill telephoned and asked to bring Mom's walker. At 5:30 p.m. on September 19, while trying to walk without her cane, Mom fell in the hallway and was taken to the hospital by ambulance. X-rays showed that she had suffered three broken ribs. After her return from the hospital, she slept through the night but the nursing notes show that Mom fell again at 6:00 a.m. on September 20, striking her head on the floor. Now her face was bruised along the entire left side and her left eye was swollen shut.

Another week went by. Though Mom had been given an antibiotic for her urinary tract infection, she continued to be delirious much of the time. About two and a half weeks after her admission, her records show that she was anemic, had an electrolyte imbalance, and was "thought," because of her delirium, to have a continuing urinary tract infection. Her serum sodium levels were also elevated, indicating dehydration. None of these conditions was treated. The other profound and ultimately fatal medical conditions, all untreated, developed thereafter.

Critically, the diagnosis of psychosis and a few days later dementia with psychosis permitted the facility to give Mom an antipsychotic, even though the Omnibus Budget Reconciliation Act (OBRA) rules described later in this chapter were not followed. There was no documentation, for example, that the facility attempted to use any method to keep Mom from harming herself or a third party without using drugs. Nor was there any documentation that the facility had made an effort to determine whether Mom's "assaultive behavior" was transitory or permanent. Despite OBRA requirements that psychotropic medications be tapered or discontinued, this did not happen either. Even when, on September 29, the discharge summary from the mental health unit stated that Mom was "considered to be significantly improved at the time of discharge as not reporting any overt psychotic symptoms," the antipsychotic was not withdrawn. When, in fact, Mom became physically incapable of walking or raising her arms, when she'd lost her ability to talk, when the dystonic side effects of the antipsychotic twisted her neck muscles so much that her head was actually lying on her right shoulder, the facility still did not discontinue the drug.

Imagine my sorrow when I reviewed Mom's medical records after her death and learned that she had asked to telephone me on the day she supposedly assaulted the staff member. Her records show that at 2:30 a.m. on September 19 she told a nurse, "I want to call my daughter in Traverse City. She's a lawyer and she'll get me out of here."

Mom was refused a telephone. She was told that she'd be advised when she could use a telephone. This never happened. As usual, I called her that afternoon and her records show that we talked for 45 minutes. By then, her terror had abated. She was confused and rambling, but she did not ask me to come and get her.

—▣—

Delirium: A Commonly Overlooked but Dangerous Problem

As a caregiver, you should be particularly alert to any sudden onset of confusion in your elderly loved one because delirium is often undiagnosed. As I will explain later in this chapter, when delirium is undiagnosed, then the critical conditions causing it are often untreated and can be fatal. Look at delirium as a kind of "fire alarm." When you suspect delirium, you will want to sound the alarm and get the first responders on the scene. Because your loved one is probably not cared for by a geriatrician, use your special knowledge about delirium—what I'm going to teach you here—to advocate for a proper diagnosis and for diagnosis of its underlying cause.

A doctor or nurse trained in geriatric medicine will normally associate an unusual confused state in a sick elderly person with delirium and will naturally understand that treatment of the underlying condition will make the delirium subside. But because most doctors and nurses are not trained in geriatrics, many do not understand the sudden onset of confusion as delirium. This can lead to misdiagnosis. If, as occurred with my mother, the doctor misdiagnoses it as dementia and fails to detect and treat the underlying medical condition, a not infrequent result is the patient's decline, or worse, her death.

Death May Result from Undiagnosed Delirium

15 to 26% of all nursing home residents who become delirious die, usually as a result of an untreated underlying disease process that is causing the delirium.

Once a diagnosis of delirium is made, it's crucial to determine the cause of it. Many treatable diseases and conditions can cause delirium. Many medications commonly prescribed for the elderly also can cause delirium. Eliminating the medication or reducing the dosage may resolve the problem. Because 15 to 26% of all nursing home residents who become delirious die, usually as a result of an untreated underlying disease process that is causing the delirium, it is imperative that a correct diagnosis be made.[2] While it is not uncommon for the elderly to suffer from confusion or forgetfulness, it is important to note that *every medical journal article I have read* concerning the diagnosis and treatment of delirium states clearly and emphatically that any acute or sudden change in an elderly person's perception and understanding of reality, consciousness, or both, *should be considered delirium until proved otherwise.* Delirium is a symptom that something is seriously wrong—that there is an underlying cause that can usually be resolved if prompt intervention occurs.

Unfortunately, dementia, delirium, and depression are the most commonly missed diagnoses in older adults with behavioral symptoms.[3] The frequency with which delirium is missed is alarming! In 1994, Dr. P. T. Tzepacz found that doctors missed a diagnosis of delirium in 95% of patients! (They missed a diagnosis of dementia in 72% of patients and missed a diagnosis of depression in 85% of patients.) In another study of hospitalized elderly patients, he found that only 5% of the deliriums were detected by physicians, despite the fact that the nursing notes contained sufficient information to diagnose delirium 85% of the time. (Dr. Tzepacz found that physicians only used the nursing notes about 20% of the time.[4]) Thus, physicians were overlooking a key source of information about changes in their patient's behavior that might have helped them make a correct diagnosis.

A primary reason why doctors miss the diagnosis so often is that they see only a fraction of resident/patient behaviors. Since physicians typically have so little actual contact with patients, the best insight into behavioral symptoms that could trigger a diagnosis of delirium, dementia, or depression comes from the people—the nurses, aides, or family members—who have the greatest opportunity to see these behaviors.

Consequently, to protect your loved one from unnecessary or inappropriate treatment of what are viewed as problem behaviors or what may be written off as psychiatric illnesses or normal effects of aging (senility), is essential that you participate in the history-taking process and that you share your unique understanding of your loved one's usual mental status to make certain the physician and nursing home facility have adequately and accurately assessed your loved one's confusion.

Ask yourself the following questions:

Is your loved one suffering from:
delirium (confusion/hallucinations, usually due to an underlying medical condition),
dementia (a chronic, progressive illness characterized by loss of memory and a severe reduction in all aspects of mental functioning), or
psychosis (a psychiatric illness or disorder)?
Has her decline in normal cognitive ability been rapid or gradual?
Has her decline been acute or does it appear to be chronic and progressive?

SUDDEN ONSET OF CONFUSION IS
THE HALLMARK OF DELIRIUM

The abrupt change in mental status is a key to identifying delirium. The onset of delirium is so sudden, usually occurring in a matter of hours to days, that it is generally possible for a family caregiver to identify a precise date when it began. The intimate knowledge you have of your loved one's normal personality and demeanor makes you the most valuable member of the caregiving team because you will usually notice significant changes long before a nurse or an aide, and you can alert them that a physician should investigate the cause of these changes in status.

Differentiating between the mental state of the patient today and the normal mental state of the patient is crucial to the diagnosis of delirium. Ideally, of course, a patient will be seen and evaluated by a physician who is familiar with her. Once an abnormal mental state is noted, the lab tests showing a urinary tract infection or other medical complication may clearly indicate delirium as the cause for a patient's agitated mental condition.

COMMON CHARACTERISTICS OF DELIRIUM

In order to help your loved one's physicians detect delirium, you'll need to know what to look for. Delirium is characterized by a sudden change in mental status resulting in confusion and disorientation, especially as to time and sometimes as to identity. A delirious person acts very much like someone who is becoming increasingly intoxicated.

Incoherent thoughts and ramblings are also common symptoms of delirium. Delirious people often see strange and frightening hallucinations. Paranoia is often experienced in delirium, and a patient may think that strange things are happening either to them or to their loved ones.

Delirium can persist from hours to days or even longer, and its severity will depend on the underlying medical circumstances. It will also depend on whether any underlying condition is properly diagnosed and treated.

Typically, delirium is characterized by the following features:

- Confusion and disorientation. These conditions are readily apparent. Patients may, however, have periods of lucidity and their mental status may fluctuate throughout the day.
- Change in attention span. Patients are no longer functional but instead have extremely short attention spans.

- Noticeable changes in patients' sleep-wake cycles. These may vary from hour to hour. Sometimes delirium is worse at night, a situation called "sundowning."
- Insomnia. This is also a common feature of delirium. In addition, some delirious people become very quiet and withdrawn, making it difficult to diagnose a problem. Other delirious people become agitated. These people may attempt to fight their hallucinations or delusions.[5]
- Drastic changes in patients' physical activities. Patients may either become lethargic and move very little or, in stark contrast, become hyperactive.[6]

MEDICAL CONDITIONS THAT COMMONLY CAUSE DELIRIUM

Knowing what can cause delirium can help you recognize it. The tests for common precipitators of delirium not only help in diagnosing delirium, but also in identifying and treating its underlying cause. Dr. Espino and his colleagues, writing for the Journal of the American Family Physician, recommend that when an acute change in mental status is observed, delirium should be suspected first and ruled out. Since delirium is so often caused by an underlying medical problem that, undetected, could lead to death, diagnostic tests should be undertaken to determine or to rule out an underlying medical condition as the cause of delirium. According to the *Merck Manual*, countless conditions or disorders can cause delirium, including readily treatable conditions such as an electrolyte imbalance, drug reactions, or serious infections.[7]

Some of the common causes of delirium in elderly people are as follows:[8]

- Urinary tract infections and the fever that persists
- Other types of infections, especially those accompanied by fever
- Side effects of many different types of medications commonly taken by elderly people for several different kinds of concurrent illnesses[9]
- Interactions between one medication and another
- A disorder of metabolism
- An electrolyte imbalance, even a minor one
- An imbalance in the levels of acids and bases in the body
- Dehydration
- Loss of the body's ability to maintain normal temperature (hypothermia)

- Retention of urine
- Fecal impaction (constipation)
- Acute blood loss
- Congestive heart failure
- Kidney failure
- The change from a familiar environment such as home to a strange environment such as a nursing home
- Under-nutrition or malnutrition
- Acute grief such as that due to the loss of a spouse or other loved one
- Substance abuse, either active or in the past
- Poor heart or lung function that leads to decreased oxygen or increased CO_2 in the blood
- Poor or non-ambulatory status (wheelchair-bound or bed-bound)
- A history of serious brain trauma such as a subdural hematoma caused by a fall or disease
- A complication after surgery in the postoperative stage
- An overload of anticholinergic drugs

Anticholinergic Medications

Many of the prescription drugs used in the treatment of Parkinson's disease, depression, allergies, migraine, and irritable bowel syndrome are anticholinergic drugs, as are some pain relieving (analgesic) drugs. Non-prescription drugs of this type are becoming increasingly available, including cold and flu medicines, indigestion tablets, sleeping pills, and anti-diarrhea treatments. The risk of side effects from a dose of one of these might be very small, but many elderly patients take several kinds of medications at once, increasing the likelihood of an "anticholinergic load." The typical side effects of anticholinergics are dry mouth, constipation, urinary problems, dizziness, likelihood of falling, anxiety, rapid shallow breathing, and irregular or rapid heartbeat.

The lab tests physicians may order when ruling out delirium and identifying its cause include: (a) a complete blood count, (b) an electrolyte test, (c) metabolic screening tests, (d) thyroid function tests, (e) Vitamin B_{12} and folate tests, (f) screening for drug toxicity, (g) tests for syphilis and HIV, (h) a urinalysis, (i) an electrocardiogram, and (j) a CT scan or MRI imaging study.[10] Physicians will test for the most common causes first, and will only order expensive tests like CT scans or MRI imaging if the earlier tests do not reveal a cause or causes of the delirium. See Appendix C for a more complete description of the tests and conditions each test is intended to detect.

MEDICATIONS: THE SECOND MOST COMMON CAUSE OF DELIRIUM

Clinicians are equally adamant that, upon ruling out a medical problem as a cause of delirium, an adverse drug reaction should be suspected. In Mom's case, the delirium caused by her urinary tract infection was exacerbated soon thereafter by the prescription of an inappropriate drug.

As will be discussed later, an elderly patient frequently suffers from more than one disease or condition and typically takes several medications as a result. Sometimes one of those medications will interact with another. The onset of delirium may help alert you and your loved one's doctors to a medication error or adverse reaction. Thus, ruling out delirium as a side effect of a medication is critical. Ordinarily, if a medication is causing delirium, eliminating the medication will resolve the delirium.

The medications most often implicated in causing delirium are:[11]

* Anticholinergic agents found in many common medications such as over-the-counter cold and allergy medicines and also in many prescription medications
* Benzodiazepines (Some common examples of these antianxiety medications include Valium, Xanax, and Ativan)
* Cardiovascular agents (some medications used to treat heart arrhythmias, for example)
* Xanthine (caffeine)
* Narcotic and nonnarcotic analgesics (some pain killers)
* Over-the-counter medications (e.g., antihistamines and anticholinergics)

Distinguishing Delirium from Dementia

You'll need to know enough about conditions that could be confused with delirium to help your loved one's physician make a proper diagnosis. If I had known then what I know now, I'd have realized that Mom's initial diagnosis of dementia—the one that resulted in her being placed in the psychiatric unit—was completely wrong. Dementia, unlike delirium, begins gradually rather than abruptly so it will be difficult at best for the family or nursing home staff to pinpoint its onset. It should be hard for the informed family caregiver to confuse delirium with dementia. Although there is an obvious change in mental status that gradually results in loss of memory and a severe decline in all aspects of mental functioning, dementia, unlike delirium, is not an acute and short-lived disease; it is a chronic illness that progresses and worsens over the years. The patient who has dementia will gradually lose the ability to perform the usual activities of daily living.

Since most dementias are incurable and patients with dementia rarely "get better," delirium as well as psychiatric disorders such as depression and/or psychosis should be ruled out before dementia is considered as a cause of a patient's confusion.

Most dementias are a result of such conditions as Alzheimer's disease, vascular dementia, central nervous system (CNS) trauma, Parkinson's disease, or far less commonly, Pick's disease, human immunodeficiency virus (HIV) infection, Creutzfeldt-Jakob disease, and Huntington's disease. Instead of using drugs, the best treatment for dementia is often a supportive environment and simplification of daily routines.

Reversible Dementia

There are some commonly recognized causes of reversible dementia such as dysfunction of the thyroid gland, vitamin deficiencies, especially B_{12} and folate, neurosyphilis and other infections, and metabolic abnormalities.

To help you identify it, consider these characteristics of dementia:

- Memory loss. The patient's confusion generally remains stable from day to day, unless an infection or other cause induces the onset of concurrent delirium.
- Physiological changes. These changes are less prominent in a patient with dementia than in one with delirium. Until the patient reaches a terminal stage in her illness, the level of consciousness is not clouded. There is not usually a marked reduction in the attention span. The patient experiences disturbances in her sleep-wake cycle, but the difficulty is seen in a reversal of night and day, not variability from hour to hour. Likewise, changes in the patient's psychomotor functions usually occur late in the dementia patient unless there is an occurrence of depression.

Distinguishing Delirium from Depression

Depression must also be distinguished from delirium. In addition to experiencing a change in function such as a depressed mood or a loss of interest in what normally brings pleasure, depressed people typically exhibit five or more of the following types of symptoms over a two-week period:[12]

- Significant changes in appetite or weight (gain or loss)
- Changes in sleep patterns (insomnia or extended sleep periods)
- Changes in psychomotor skills (too active or not active)
- A loss in energy; obvious fatigue
- Expressions of feelings of guilt or lack of worth
- Changes in the ability to think logically, to concentrate, or to make decisions
- Thoughts of death, or a compromised ability to function at prior levels
- Thoughts of suicide, or attempts or plans to commit suicide
- Lack of alternative reasons for a depressed mood such as a natural grief reaction
- Lack of a medical condition or substance abuse to account for the depression
- Prominent distress and a compromised ability to function at prior levels

If depression is a cause of behavior problems, there are approved medications to treat the condition, though antidepressants typically have been under-utilized since depression is often overlooked as a cause of behavioral disturbances in the elderly.[13]

Distinguishing Delirium from Psychosis

There are marked differences between delirium and psychosis, the latter being a psychiatric illness or disorder involving impaired reality testing, delusions, or hallucinations. According to the *Merck Manual*, the differences between the two conditions are as follows:

> A delirious patient is commonly confused about the current time, date, location, or even her identity. A psychotic patient, on the other hand, is commonly aware of these facts.

A delirious patient usually will have difficulty paying attention; the opposite is usually true of the psychotic patient.

Short-term memory loss characterizes delirium. A psychotic patient, on the contrary, may think illogically but usually experiences no short-term memory loss.

A delirious patient usually is unable to think logically or to perform even simple calculations while the psychotic patient retains those abilities.

While the delirious patient usually has a fever and/or other signs of infection, the psychotic patient does not.

The psychotic patient often has a history of previous mental illness; the delirious patient often does not.

The delirious patient may be preoccupied with various concerns or worries but is usually inconsistent in her worrying tendencies. By contrast, a psychotic patient will often be fixated on concerns that are consistently the same.

Both patients will experience hallucinations, but the delirious patient's hallucinations will usually be visual while the psychotic patient's will be auditory.

Tremor is another common sign of delirium and is not a symptom of psychosis.[14] Unfortunately, tremor is also a symptom of Parkinson's disease, and medical personnel are well aware that psychosis is a common condition in last-stage Parkinson's patients. This makes an inappropriate diagnosis of psychosis credible in a patient with Parkinson's disease.

Psychotropic Medications and Delirium

As I mentioned earlier, once Mom was admitted to the psychiatric unit, her bizarre hallucinations and her confusion quickly resulted in the prescription of a dangerous antipsychotic medication. Mom's earlier diagnosis of Parkinson's disease may have been a reason why this medication was prescribed, for psychosis often develops in the later stages of Parkinson's disease. But because the physician directing Mom's care at this stage of the game was not experienced in geriatrics or in treating PD, he made a critical error in choosing this drug, as I will explain in Chapter Three. You will need to know certain facts to help your loved one's physician avoid making a similar error, especially if she lives in a nursing home.

Dr. Mark Beers and his colleagues have been at the forefront of the campaign to avoid the use of psychotropic medications in the elderly.[15] In spite of their efforts, psychotropic drugs are often used with nursing home residents diagnosed with dementia to "cure" behavior seen as inappropriate, such as "wandering" and agitation. This is true even though (a) there is no evidence that antipsychotics will improve dementia, (b) psychotropic medications do not halt the progression of dementia, and (c) federal law prohibits the use of psychotropic medications in nursing home residents diagnosed with dementia unless psychosis is a diagnosed component of the condition.

Sadly, despite attempts at federal oversight, nursing homes continue to advocate for what are truly chemical restraints. In a newsletter sent to nursing homes by the government agency in charge of oversight, pharmacologist Thomas Snader wrote that antipsychotics are usually useless in controlling problem behaviors and carry significant risk of toxicity, including serious side effects.[16]

Antipsychotics Frequently Prescribed in Nursing Homes

Martin T. Miller Associates, a health care data collection and consulting firm, reports that total sales of medications for nursing facility residents for the 12 months ending June 30, 1997, were $1,387,399,640. The drug at the top of the list was the antipsychotic implicated in my mom's death.

Given the caution of these physicians and others, it is truly amazing that antipsychotics represent the most prescribed (dollar-wise) of all medications used in nursing homes![17] In fact, studies have found that most residents of long-term care facilities at some time during their stay receive at least one psychotropic medication.[18] In 50 to 75% of the elderly, antipsychotic-induced side effects and extrapyramidal symptoms (EPSs) will cause serious problems[19] that are examined at length in Chapter Four.

By helping the medical staff analyze troublesome behaviors of your loved one, you may be able to prevent your loved one's exposure to these drugs. With very limited exceptions, as you will learn below, antipsychotics should almost never be prescribed for a delirious patient; these drugs should likewise rarely be prescribed for the patient with dementia. As I learned while caring for Mom and also later when doing the research for this book, family caregivers need to be aware of the dangers and also of their right to advocate with medical caregivers to avoid use of these drugs.

PROTECTING YOUR LOVED ONE FROM DANGEROUS PSYCHOTROPIC DRUGS

If your loved one is prescribed a psychotropic drug, I urge you to investigate thoroughly. You will want to look at her records to verify that the federal regulations controlling the use of these dangerous medications have been followed. See Appendix Q. In fact, this may be one of the times when you will insist upon consultation with a geriatrician so that you can avoid the potential for serious consequences.

We were told that our mother could not see her own internist because that doctor was "not approved" to practice in the nursing home where Mom was a resident. We could, however, have made an appointment for our mom with her own doctor and taken her from the nursing home to that appointment. I remain confident that Mom's doctor would have been very struck by the dramatic change in Mom's physical and mental condition and that she would have recognized the significance of the sudden onset of confusion that doctors who were strangers to her did not appreciate. We might then have had a medical opinion that confirmed that the dangerous drug Mom was given should be eliminated. That would have reduced her tremor and the difficulty in swallowing that led to her subsequent medical difficulties, and it might have made all the difference.

What You Can Do to Help Your Loved One's Physician Detect Delirium

Maintain a History. In Chapter Four, you will learn how to put together a three-ring binder that lists each illness and medication your loved one has. You will also learn how to establish a baseline for her medical condition, mental acuity, and physical condition. Using this written record of your loved one's status together with regular observations of her, you will be able to assess changes in status and should be readily able to determine whether she is suffering from delirium, dementia, or psychosis. You can use the checklist in Appendix D to identify risk factors your loved one has that might lead to delirium.

Use the checklist in Appendix E to identify physiological causes of behavior that should not trigger the prescription of a psychotropic medication for her. For example, one clinician wrote about a female nursing home resident who sat in her wheelchair screaming for most of the day, an unusual behavior for that particular patient. In some facilities, constant screaming would trigger the automatic prescription of a medication, often one that could be harmful to the resident such as an inappropriate antipsychotic. In this case, however, a staff member finally noticed that the woman's finger was caught in the mechanism of her wheelchair. Thus, it was possible to rule out delirium, to prevent the prescription of an unnecessary drug, to free the woman's finger from its painful situation, and to attend to her pain and her injury!

Advocate for Your Loved One's Treatment. If you maintain regular contact with your loved one, you will be in a good position to act as an advocate for her. Keep in mind that you are a member of a team and that overwork, tension, and other countless stressors are a part of the larger picture. An adversarial tone may alienate her caregivers or make them defensive. Think in terms of building alliances and make it clear that you are working with her caregivers, not against them. You will want to maintain your composure as a team player, never bullying or harassing other caregivers. It is clear that many horrible results have occurred in some care facilities, but it would be a mistake to assume that the worst will happen. No one wants your loved one to have a bad result. Therefore, by maintaining respectful communications with her caregivers while avoiding becoming part of the problem, you'll be in a position to be a part of the solution.

You can advocate for your loved one's treatment in the following ways:

Rule Out Delirium. Request that delirium be ruled out first and be certain that all possible diagnostics are done. This means you will have to look at all potential causes for the confusion your loved one is experiencing—an underlying illness, medications, or physiological reasons—in light of the facts you have gathered. If you suspect delirium, check her medical chart to determine whether any recent laboratory results exist. Ask her physician about abnormal results.

You can also ask your loved one's physician to order a full physical examination. The physician should observe the resident's neurologic responses. She may order laboratory tests to detect infections, metabolic or electrolyte disorders, and other measurable diseases or conditions that can cause delirium. X-rays may be ordered to confirm or deny the existence of a subdural hematoma. A spinal tap may be ordered to detect infection. A neurological work-up that includes an EEG (electroencephalogram) may help to make a diagnosis. Obviously, if a previous EEG is available for comparison, this will be very helpful. Last, a CT scan or MRI may detect brain trauma or other changes in the brain. Note that these diagnostic tools are used in an order intended to detect first the most common conditions that may be the root cause of her change in status. The latter tests are used to find the less common disorders. Often the cause of your loved one's distress will be found earlier and thus not all diagnostics will be used.

Evaluate Medications As a Possible Cause of Delirium. Request that all current medications be evaluated to determine whether a drug reaction caused by too many drugs being taken is the root cause of the confusion. Again, the following types of prescription drugs are most often implicated as causing delirium: anticholinergic agents, benzodiazepines, cardiovascular agents, xanthine (caffeine), and both narcotic and nonnarcotic analgesics.[20] Over-the-counter medications such as antihistamines and anticholinergics can also cause delirium.[21]

Advocate for Non-Pharmaceutical Interventions. Request that non-pharmaceutical interventions be considered first in any attempts to modify behavior. These interventions usually include various changes in the resident's environment such as using music to calm a resident who is experiencing auditory hallucinations or using low-wattage lights to calm a resident who is experiencing visual hallucinations.[22]

Ensure a Proper Assessment for Delirium. Request that proper assessment and documentation of a perceived need for the prescription of a psychoactive medication be done and made available for your review prior to the administration of any medication. Because of the dangers these medications pose for your loved one, you'll want to verify that she has an appropriate assessment, which could include, at a minimum, the following:

- A chart review to determine whether changes in her drug regimen, occurrences of recent falls, trauma, infections, or delirium due to dehydration, constipation, lack of glycemic control, imbalances of her electrolytes or metabolic system, or neurological problems could be the root cause of the change in behavior.
- A chart review to determine whether recent changes in her medications or physical discomfort could be the cause of the change in behavior.
- A careful assessment of her current medications to determine whether an adverse drug reaction could be the cause of her delirium.

- The laboratory tests described in Appendix C to rule out a newly developed medical condition as the cause or exacerbation of her delirium.
- An assessment to determine whether visual impairment or environmental problems, including stress or grief, could be a cause of the change in behavior.
- A qualitative and quantitative assessment of her need for interventions of any kind, pharmaceutical or not. In other words, how serious is the altered behavior and how often does it occur? Such an assessment could also include a determination of whether the presenting behaviors are transient or permanent.

Refuse Antipsychotics. Your loved one has the right to refuse any treatment, including the use of antipsychotics. If you are her patient advocate and have the legal authority to make her health care decisions, you also have the right to insist that these drugs not be used or, if they have already been prescribed, that they be discontinued.

As you'll read in a later chapter, Mom might have survived if I'd followed through on my request that the antipsychotic be discontinued. Instead, it never occurred to me to check. The drug continued to be used right up until the day before I transferred her, despite the fact that by then she was bed-ridden and unable to raise herself, let alone a cane.

It may be foreign to your nature to be assertive, but as your loved one's advocate, you should strive to prevent the use of these powerful, potentially harmful, and usually useless drugs.

Remain Actively Involved in Assessment and Treatment Options. How your loved one's physician treats delirium will depend upon the underlying cause. Infections, for example, will be treated with antibiotics; abnormal salt and mineral levels in the blood will be treated by regulating levels of fluids and salts. Your loved one's medications may be modified if the cause of the delirium is a reaction to one or more drugs in her current drug regimen. That very issue, medication errors, is addressed in the following chapter.

CHAPTER THREE

Silent Epidemic: Types and Frequency of Medication Errors in the Elderly

SEPTEMBER 29, 2000

Glen and I left home at about 10:00 in the morning. Mom was being transferred today from the behavioral medicine unit of Alpine Manor to its skilled nursing unit and we were going downstate to see her. We arrived at the nursing home at about 2:00 in the afternoon. As we walked to the building from the parking lot, we met Kris, Mom's eldest grandson, walking toward us. He was going to buy some playing cards. Kris and his sister, Trisha, had flown from Florida to see their "Nana" and spend the weekend visiting with her.

We went up to the fifth floor, the medical unit. Jill had brought in Mom's walker and there we found Trisha helping Nana walk around the unit to become familiar with this new environment. Mom's ribs were healing, and though her face was still colored from the fall she'd had on September 19, her bruises had turned greenish-yellow.

We ended up in the common room and found a table where we could play cards. I later learned that residents of a nursing home, as required by OBRA, have the right to a private area in which to visit with family, friends, and others. No one offered us a private area on this day, and it was very noisy in the solar-ium with the large TV blaring away, although fewer than half of the residents were watching it.

Mom was glad to see everyone. Although she seemed a little weak, she was otherwise our mom. She had been in the facility nearly two weeks, and though her delirium would soon return because the antibiotic she was prescribed had not cured her urinary tract infection, we observed no confusion or delirium at this time. On the contrary, she was alert and ready to socialize. We played euchre, as Kris had arrived with pinochle decks instead of full decks of cards. Because there were five of us, one of us sat out each game. Mom's bidding was a little more daring than I'd remembered it, but she and her partner won every game but one of the five or six we played.

Mom's dinner came and we quit playing while she ate. She was obviously hungry and she finished her dinner. When the physical therapist came to talk with her about a PT plan, Mom handed me her cards to play while she independently gave the therapist her history and planned her therapy. Because Mom had fallen numerous times in the past two weeks, the medical director had ordered physical therapy for her.

The tough part was when we prepared to leave, five hours later at about 7:00 p.m. Mom knew that we were all going to her house for dinner with Jill and she started to weep. She just couldn't bear the thought of not being with all of us for dinner. Mom did not yet have a TV package so she had no TV in her room. The room had four beds, and the woman in the corner was loudly and constantly moaning. Mom was truly upset and it was just awful to have to leave her there.

Finally, a nurse came in and said that she would try to find a TV controller for Mom. She also said that a room had opened up down the hall and that she could move the woman who was filling the room with incoherent moaning. We promised Mom that we would bring some asparagus and salmon to her the next morning so that she could have for lunch what we were having for dinner.

Mom finally calmed down and we left. At dinner, we celebrated Jill's birthday. However, there was little cheer among the five of us as we contemplated what lay ahead for our mom and nana.

The following day, Glen and I visited with Mom in the morning. Later, Kris and Trisha's father, Dan, visited with her for about an hour. She shared with him the photographs we'd brought to her showing parts of the hot air balloon ride we'd had the week before. Trisha and Kris spent about seven hours with Nana that day. When we all talked about the weekend later, we remembered that Nana was almost her old self—almost, but still in need of physical therapy so that she could regain some of her former stability and mobility.

OCTOBER, 2000

Over the next two weeks, I began to search for an adult foster care home (AFCH) for Mom in or near Traverse City. Because of her delirium and the numerous falls, it was apparent that Mom's home was not an appropriate place for her. No one was home during the daytime and Mom needed someone to watch over her. I started with an AFCH run by an old friend of mine. Mom knew Martha and had actually been in her home for dinner and cards years before. Martha ran her adult foster care home like a bed and breakfast and I thought Mom would be very comfortable there. It would not be optimally convenient for me, as it was 45 miles from our home, but I felt that Mom would *more easily make the transition from independent living to living in a care-giving facility because of the ties with Martha and also because of the small, intimate nature of the home.*

First Martha said yes, that she could care for Mom. Two days later, my hopes were dashed when she telephoned to say she'd changed her mind—that she'd only said yes because of our friendship. Martha told me how difficult it had been for her to find and keep aides and how she had been trying to sell her business for the past year or so. She did not want to accept another resident.

I next telephoned the local office of the Family Independence Agency, the state agency that licenses foster care and adult foster care homes in Michigan. Several days later, I received a packet from them listing all of the AFCHs in our four-county area. Then, after I'd had time to review it, I received a telephone call from a consultant with the agency. I described Mom's physical, mental, and medical condition. I also described her social interests. I was particularly interested in finding an AFCH where the other residents would be ladies with similar interests and abilities. I also was interested in finding one close to our home so that I could pick Mom up and take her to bridge games or to lunch and bring her to our house on weekends. With this information, the consultant was able to guide me toward about a dozen facilities that she knew had openings.

The next step was to telephone each of the AFCHs to inquire about vacancies, costs, and to schedule visits.

During this time, I talked to Mom on the telephone every day. On about the sixth day of October, I noticed that Mom was again confused. She began again to describe terrifying incidents involving members of our family, usually grandchildren. She imagined everything from job-related fatalities to house fires. I would listen to her news and then gently say, "No, Mom, that was just another bad dream."

During October, Kris and Trisha were also talking to Nana on the phone and Jill and Betsy were visiting every day. Emails went back and forth between Florida, Saginaw, and Traverse City. We were all concerned about Mom's lapse back into her hallucinations. Jill said that the nurses had told her that Mom had another urinary tract infection.

When Mom began to have trouble talking, we again were alarmed. Kris and Trisha both emailed me to ask why Nana was incoherent on the telephone. Jill and I talked with the nurses. Their common reply to our concerns was, "This is to be expected."

OCTOBER 15, 2000

I drove to Saginaw to see Mom and also to meet with Jill and go to the University of Michigan Hospital to consult with Jill's physicians. I met Jill at Alpine

Manor and we went together to Mom's room. She'd been transferred again—this time to the fourth floor. These many transfers further undermined Mom's treatment: she was never in one unit long enough for the staff to be able to get to know her or to adequately detect or assess changes in her status.

Jill told me that Mom's transfer had been explained as a lateral move and that Mom would continue to receive physical therapy. The difference, Jill said, was that the physical therapist would come to Mom instead of Mom going to the basement PT room.

We learned after Mom's death that the real reason Mom was transferred was that her Medicare had run out. She would now be covered by Medicaid, which pays the facility less, so she was being transferred from skilled nursing to an extended care unit.

Mom was sitting in a wheelchair in the solarium when we arrived. I was surprised to see this, as she had been walking on September 29. The nurses explained that Mom was too unsteady on her feet and, also, that she usually failed to ask for assistance in getting up. Numerous falls made it safer for her to be in a wheelchair. She also had an alarm clipped on her blouse so that the nurses would be alerted if she tried to get up without help.

At first glance, Mom seemed asleep, her chin resting on her chest. When I spoke to her, she raised her head. The first words she said were, "I have to go to the bathroom." Jill and I grew accustomed to Mom's request for toileting assistance at the beginning of each visit. We were not sure if Mom was too shy to ask the aides for help or if the aides simply ignored her needs. We did not consider that her difficulty with toileting might lead her to decrease her fluid intake, nor did we understand the dangers that posed for her.

Jill and I found an aide to assist Mom in the lavatory. I noticed that she was far more unstable today than she had been two weeks earlier. The ability to stand or to walk unassisted that she had shown two weeks before was gone.

To have more privacy, we went with her to her room. It was pleasant enough, a double. Mom had the bed by the window and the other bed was empty. I had brought Mom a book of bridge strategy and also a box of bridge hands clipped from the newspaper. I'd developed the habit of saving the bridge columns for her. Because it was the only part of the newspaper she read, it seemed to make more sense for me to supply them to her from our daily paper than for her to subscribe to a paper. When I handed them to her, she got tears in her eyes. She looked at me and said tremulously, "I miss everything so much." I told her that I understood and that it must be hard not to be at home. I told her that she just needed to work with her physical therapist so that she would get stronger and improve her walking. Once she was steady on her feet again, she would leave this place.

Jill stayed and talked with Mom while I went to the nurses' station. The charge nurse and Mom's nurse were both there. I introduced myself and asked them whether Mom had been evaluated for depression. They seemed unsure about that, so I asked to see her medication sheet. I noted that medications for Parkinson's, for angina, for gastrointestinal reflux disease (GERD), and for osteoporosis were being given. I noticed another drug, the name of which I did not recognize. When I asked what the drug was for, they told me it was an antipsychotic.

The antipsychotic[1] Mom was given was prescribed, I believe, for the convenience of the nursing home staff. At the time, I didn't know that no medical study had ever approved an antipsychotic to treat delirium or dementia. I also didn't know that federal law prohibits the use of antipsychotics for delirium unless the patient exhibits psychotic and/or agitated behaviors. Unfortunately, I also did not know that antipsychotics have so many deleterious side effects for the elderly that they should be used only as a last resort or that in most cases, antipsychotics will not "cure" the problem or significantly improve the behavior.[2]

I told the nurses that Mom was not crazy, but that she undoubtedly was depressed. I described how Mom had come to be there in the first place and how she had walked into the facility only one month earlier. I described how independent and socially active she had been just one month ago. I described in detail the long afternoon of card playing and the two days of long visiting that Mom had participated in only two weeks before. I explained how she'd been walking with a walker then. Both nurses kept saying they found it hard to believe that Mom had functioned so well as recently as two to four weeks ago.

At this time, I requested that the antipsychotic be discontinued[3] and that Mom be evaluated for depression. As Mom's designated patient advocates, Jill and I under Michigan law had the absolute right in a time of Mom's disability to refuse any treatment.

Both nurses said that the medical director would be making rounds on the weekend and that they would talk with him about my request. Tragically, I did not follow up to make sure that my request was honored. Inexplicably, the facility failed to honor the request to discontinue the treatment and also failed to advise us of the medical director's decision in that regard, or to explain the reasons behind this decision.

I expressed my concerns about Mom's worsening condition. Her nurse, Michelle, told me, "Home care is the best care." She looked at me very deliberately as she said this. Looking back, I can't help but believe she was trying to give me a message, something that she could not say in front of the charge nurse. I believe she was telling me to get Mom out of there, and I can't believe I didn't understand.

OCTOBER 16, 2000

After our return from Ann Arbor, where Jill explored with her physicians the benefits and detriments of genetic testing in breast cancer patients, I dropped Jill at the house and went to Alpine Manor to see Mom. Once again, she was in the solarium, seemingly asleep in her wheelchair, chin on her chest. I gathered that the nurses put all of the residents who needed "15-minute checks" in the solarium so that they could more easily do their "checks."

I went to Mom's side. When I spoke to her, she raised her head. "I need to go to the bathroom," she said. This time, it was more difficult to find an aide to help as it was approaching dinnertime. Finally, I found an aide. I noted that she automatically took an adult diaper from a huge rack next to the door to the bathing room as she entered. There was no apparent effort at bladder and bowel control training, as is required to maintain functional status. The demoralizing effect of this loss of dignity must have been awful for Mom.

When Mom came out, I put a silvery package in her lap. "I brought you a present from Ann Arbor," I told her. Her hands were trembling more than I'd remembered. She needed help with the bright red ribbon. Inside the box was a gangly-legged bunny. It was fuzzy and white, wearing a pink sweater with huge red strawberries on it. "I thought you might like something cuddly to sleep with," I told her. Her dinner came soon. I noticed that the aide put it down in front of her and cut the pancakes into bite sizes for her.

Clearly, Mom's physical status had changed for the worse. Because of the incontinence problems and because she was wheelchair-bound, Mom was not a candidate for an AFCH. Thus, when I returned to Traverse City, I began to search for a nursing home. I did not know that I should have spent less time trying to find a new facility for her and more effort expediting the move.

—⌑—

Medication Errors

Because many common illnesses and life-threatening conditions are caused each year as a result of medication errors, you'll want to learn more about how to prevent these from harming your loved one.[4] Once you learn what to look for, you will be the person most able to alert her physicians and nurses that her medications should be reevaluated. Advocating for a reduction in medications and dosages, when needed, should be a primary focus of your caregiving.

Most medication errors have been found to occur in the prescribing—either the choice of drug or the dosage recommended. An important reason why these errors occur is that most physicians are not trained to pre-scribe for the elderly, as Dr. Friedman explained in Chapter One.

Another reason why medication errors are one of the greatest hazards to your loved one's health is the fact that many elderly have concurrent illnesses that are treated with various drugs. The prescribing of multiple different medications to one patient is known as polypharmacy, and is an increasing problem with the elderly. Quite simply, the greater the number of diseases and conditions combined with the greater the number of drugs prescribed, including over-the-counter medications, the greater the incremental risk your loved one has for drug-drug, drug-food, and/or drug-disease interactions.

The following are the eight categories of medication-related problems in patients that have been identified by Dr. Mark Beers and his colleagues:

1. **Untreated Symptoms/Illness**. The patient has a medical problem that requires drug therapy but is not receiving medication for that problem.

2. **Improper Drug Selection**. The patient has a medical problem that requires drug therapy but is being given the wrong medication—wrong because the drug conflicts with a disease, condition, or medication the patient already has.

A common medication error is the prescription of an antipsychotic for a Parkinson's disease patient, since many antipsychotics are the pharma-ceutical opposite of Parkinson's medications. Parkinson's disease results when the brain produces an insufficient amount of dopamine, an impor-tant neurotransmitter affecting motor control or movement. Medications prescribed to treat Parkinson's stimulate the production of dopamine, but many antipsychotics actually block dopamine. Consequently, such an antipsychotic may worsen the tremors of Parkinson's disease by keeping the patient's usual medication from doing its job. The potential for serious harm is compounded by the fact that most physicians and nurses will likely consider the acute symptoms, in particular an increase in tremor and gait problems, as a worsening of her PD, not as a sign that a medication error or adverse drug reaction has occurred.

Worse, as several clinicians have noted, many elderly persons may suffer from Parkinson's disease that is undiagnosed. When an antipsychotic blocks what little dopamine the patient's brain is producing, the patient's parkinsonism (characteristic tremors) will become more pronounced. It takes a while for the cumulative effects of the antipsychotic to become noticeable. Because weeks may go by between prescription of

the drug and an increase in tremors, the patient may then be diagnosed with Parkinson's disease, while the connection between the tremors
and the drug goes unrecognized and the drug-disease interaction is
undiagnosed. If this occurs, the drug may not be withdrawn to resolve
the movement disorders that have resulted from the inappropriate
medication.

A common medication error in some nursing homes is the choice of an
inappropriate antibiotic to treat a urinary tract infection (UTI). One such
antibiotic, trimethoprim-sulfamethoxazole, is a good drug and is effective
in treating UTIs in younger patients. You might know this drug by the
brand name Bactrim or Septra. It is also a relatively inexpensive antibiotic.
However, one potential side effect of this drug is dysphagia (difficulty in
swallowing), which makes trimethoprim-sulfamethoxazole inappropriate
for an elderly patient. It has other side effects that are also dangerous for
the elderly. Joel Shuster, a pharmacologist and member of the board of
trustees of the Institute for Safe Medication Practices[5] with whom I corre-
sponded in February 2001, stated that medical professionals trained in
geriatric pharmacology do not regard trimethoprim-sulfamethoxazole as a
safe antibiotic for use in the elderly. He wrote, "Many geriatricians
NEVER use trimethoprim-sulfamethoxazole in the elderly because it
has been reported to sometimes cause CNS (central nervous system)
problems—confusion, psychosis, etc."

Despite its inappropriateness, trimethoprim-sulfamethoxazole is often
prescribed in long-term care facilities because it is a far less expensive
alternative than some of the other choices. Sadly, the assessment of cost of
treatment is a critical part of any prescribing done in a nursing home. The
best drug under the circumstances may not be prescribed because it is too
expensive.

3. **Sub-Therapeutic Dosage**. The patient has a medical problem that is
being treated with an inadequate dose of the correct medication. This may
be a dosage that is too small or a drug that is prescribed for too short a
period of time. This is not usually the type the medication error that occurs
in the elderly.

4. **Failure to Receive Drugs**. The patient has a medical problem that is
the result of not receiving a drug for pharmaceutical, psychological, socio-
logical, or economic reasons. Many nursing homes lack the facilities for
doing on-site laboratory tests. Because UTIs are a common affliction in the
elderly, it is not unusual for nursing home residents and for the elderly living in their own homes to go several days with an undiagnosed and
untreated UTI or other infection.

5. **Over-Dosage**. The patient has a medical problem that is being treated with too much of the correct drug. Unfortunately, this is a frequent problem for elderly patients. What may be a normal dose for a normal adult could be an overdose for a frail elder whose kidneys are not functioning well. Most drugs are excreted through the kidneys, although some are excreted through the liver. When the kidneys are not working well, those drugs can accumulate and cause toxicity. Drug manufacturers commonly recommend that the elderly take one half the normal adult dose. Even that amount can be too much for a frail elderly person whose kidneys are functioning at one half or one quarter of what is normal for that particular patient. Up-to-date lab tests will determine how well your loved one's kidneys are functioning, information you will need when assessing her drug regimen, including proposed new drugs as well as her usual drugs.

6. **Adverse Drug Reactions (ADRs)**. The patient has a medical problem that is the result of an unintended and harmful adverse drug effect. ADRs in turn can cause drug-induced diseases. Over half of drug-induced disorders are manifested as bleeding, bone marrow suppression, central nervous system effects, and skin reactions. Holland and DeGruy, in order of most frequent to least frequent, list the following types of drug-induced disorders:

- Bone marrow suppression
- Bleeding (such as an ulcer caused by aspirin)
- Central nervous system effects (such as tremor or confusion)
- Allergic/cutaneous reactions (such as a rash or a cough)
- Metabolic effects (disorders involving body chemistry)
- Cardiac effects (such as a irregular heartbeat)
- Gastrointestinal effects (such as severe nausea and vomiting, diarrhea, and constipation)
- Kidney problems (such as complicated by dehydration)
- Respiratory effects (such as rapid shallow breathing)

The subject of ADRs is addressed fully in Chapter Four.

7. **Drug Use without Indication**. The patient is taking a drug without a valid medical reason.

8. **Drug Interactions**. The patient has a medical problem that is the result of a drug-drug, drug-food, or drug-laboratory interaction.[6]

Drug-drug interactions may take many forms. For example, a drug-drug interaction can result in a patient getting less drug than is intended. For example, calcium interferes with absorption of some antibiotics such as

Levaquin and other quinolone antibiotics, leading to lower amounts of the antibiotics getting into the bloodstream. As a result, the infection being treated may not abate.

Other drug-drug interactions include the one described earlier, the administration of an antipsychotic to a patient taking medications for Parkinson's disease. When the antipsychotic achieves the opposite result—when it blocks dopamine, a neurotransmitter essential for normal movement—it counteracts the intended beneficial result expected with a Parkinson's medication, producing a negative patient outcome.

Other drug-drug interactions may result in an additive effect. These can occur when two drugs are used concurrently that depress the central nervous system (culprits here include alcoholic beverages, some anti-anxiety medications, antipsychotics, or certain antihistamine drugs). The result will be excessive sedation and fatigue. The elderly are particularly susceptible to this type of drug-drug interaction, and to a consequent risk of falls and injuries.

The concurrent use of two or more drugs with anticholinergic activity such as certain antipsychotics, some antiparkinsonian drugs, and some antidepressants commonly results in an overload of anticholinergic effects, including dry mouth, constipation, blurred vision, and fever. Elderly patients frequently experience the additive effects of anticholinergic effects as a type of delirium, which may imitate accelerating psychiatric symptoms or dementia, increased memory impairment, and decreased ability to provide self-care. You should consider whether one of your loved one's medications is inappropriate if she experiences blurred vision, dry mouth, constipation, and fever.

Gastrointestinal bleeding in the elderly is common, often fatal, and frequently caused by medications. It is not uncommon for the elderly to take several different products that contain the same NSAID (non-steroidal anti-inflammatory drug purchased over-the-counter or by prescription for arthritis such as Motrin, Daypro, Relafen, Advil, aspirin, Excedrin, and many others). This is particularly true if they are using over-the-counter medications—for some reason, people often think these are harmless. You should carefully review your loved one's use of pain-relievers to help her avoid this serious risk.

You'll read more about common drug-drug interactions in Chapter Four. You'll also find a chart showing drug-drug interactions involving medications, both prescription and over the counter, that are commonly taken by the elderly in Appendix G.

Who Suffers Most from Medication Errors?

It should not come as a surprise that the elderly are most at risk from the effects of medication error or that medication-related problems are generally more severe in the elderly.[7] A 1996 study by the General Accounting Office found that 17.5% of the nearly 30 million Medicare recipients received medications considered to be inappropriate for that population.

Research reveals that medication errors are prevalent. A significant number of nursing home residents are hospitalized for extensive periods of time as a result of medication errors. For example, a 1990 study estimated the percentage of hospitalizations of older patients due to medication errors to be 17%.

The risk to the elderly is nearly six times greater than for the general population.[8] Most medication errors are, according to research, preventable. Tragically, many of these errors are not prevented. The following chapter takes a closer look at an insidious result of medication errors. It also examines adverse drug reactions in greater detail. Finally, it discusses how you can help your loved one's physicians and nurses prevent medication errors and adverse drug reactions.

CHAPTER FOUR

A Closer Look:
Adverse Drug Reactions and
How to Prevent Them

OCTOBER 27, 2000

Glen drove with me to Saginaw to visit with Mom. I had narrowed the search to two nursing homes. I now needed to approach Mom with the idea of moving. Glen went to run an errand while I went up to see her. I again found her in the solarium. Her chair was positioned so that she faced the nurse's station. This time, instead of her chin being on her chest, Mom was slumped in her wheelchair, her head resting on her right shoulder. She was unable to raise her head and had to peer up at me using only her eyes.

Once again, Mom's first words to me were, "I have to go to the bathroom." I found an aide. This time the aide asked me to help her. We went into the large bathing room and the nurse wheeled Mom's chair up to the sink and helped her stand up. Then she told Mom to put her hands on the sink and to support her own weight. I noted how much more unstable Mom was, how much thinner her legs seemed. She was lethargic and apathetic. I said cheerily, "Mom, did you know that yesterday was my birthday? I was 59. Next year will be another big one." Mom did not reply. This was very unlike her.

The aide put her into a different chair and wheeled her over to a toilet. The chair slid over the toilet bowl. The aide indicated that I should turn on the water in the sink. I did this, remembering that running water was the stimulus I'd used with my babies to get them to use the toilet. After Mom voided, the aide put another adult diaper on her. Her loss of continence surprised and dismayed me.

I approached the nurses. "What is wrong with Mom's neck?" I asked. They didn't know. I asked whether an X-ray had been done to determine whether there was something wrong with her neck. They didn't think so. I asked them to find Mom a wheelchair that would provide her with support for her neck. They said they would try.

They also said that they'd talk to her physician about her neck. Later, I would discover that, in violation of federal law, Mom's "attending physician" never once saw Mom in all the time she was at Alpine Manor.

Glen was now with me. For the first time, the nurses offered us the conference room so that we could have a private visit. I talked to Mom about my search for a nursing home. I asked her if she would be willing to go to Traverse City to live so that she could be nearer to us and so that we could oversee her care. Mom was not entirely happy about this decision, but she was willing to do as I asked. She was a little uncertain about cold winters in our more northerly clime. I assured her that I'd make sure she had everything she needed to stay warm.

I also asked her if she trusted me enough to allow me to be her guardian and she agreed to this as well. Although as her patient advocate I had the legal authority to make treatment decisions for Mom if she were unable to participate in them, as a legal guardian, all treatment decisions would be mine. Many nursing homes pressure families to establish legal guardianships through the court system and, in fact, the admissions director of the Traverse City nursing home I was looking at had suggested this in my initial conference with her.

A major advantage to a guardianship is that if a resident becomes mentally or physically disabled and cannot make health care decisions, there is no delay in the providing of necessary services if the guardian agrees with staff recommendations. A major disadvantage to a legal guardianship is that there is a loss of autonomy for the resident. It is difficult to undo a guardianship. A guardianship requires a great level of trust between the elder and the person chosen to function as the guardian.

After our discussion, I found the playing cards and Glen and I started to play euchre with Mom. We both noted that she was not alert. She was trying very hard to play with us, to act like her old self, but she fumbled trying to hold five cards in her hand. She had a hard time getting the cards to the table and she was obviously having a hard time concentrating on the game. We played to five points, then Mom said that she'd had enough.

I assured her that we would have her moved in about a week and told her that I was waiting for a decision from one of two nursing homes about whether they had a vacancy for her. We left, deeply concerned about Mom's obviously deteriorating health.

Later, when I described this visit to Jill, she would tell me that both she and Betsy, who visited Mom every day, found it amazing that we were able to have a conversation with Mom, let alone play cards with her.

NOVEMBER 1, 2000
Glen and I were back in Saginaw and I'd made arrangements with the social worker on Mom's floor to be present with a notary public today. I had a petition

for guardianship with me. After Mom signed it, the petition would be granted without Mom having to be present at the hearing. Because I wanted to make sure there was no question about her competency, I'd asked for these two witnesses to her signature.

When I got to Mom's floor, I looked for her in the solarium. When I could not find her, I asked her nurse where she was. Michelle took me to Mom's room.

Mom was curled up asleep on her bed. It was one o'clock in the afternoon.

Michelle roused Mom and helped her to rise slowly to a sitting position. She explained to me that Mom was experiencing orthostatic hypotension, dizziness, if she stood up too rapidly. This was caused by her medications, Michelle said. I watched Michelle help Mom to her feet. She was trying to maneuver Mom into her wheelchair. I wondered why Mom was having so much trouble moving her feet. Utterly uncoordinated, they seemed to drag on the floor.

It would not be until long after Mom's death, after I had researched for weeks and months, that I would recognize all of the many signs of medication errors that had gone unnoticed by the nurses and Mom's physician. After I'd used a medical dictionary to look up the terms used to name side effects and adverse drug reactions given in the package insert, I would realize that Mom's shuffling gait was called "bradykinesia" and was just one of the many side effects of the antipsychotic.

But bradykinesia was not the most deadly side effect Mom experienced. Once again, I was alarmed to see her head resting on her right shoulder. After her death, my research revealed that this was a "dystonia," a particularly dangerous problem because it contributed to Mom's inability to eat, drink, or speak. When I talked to Mom, she'd move her eyes, peering up at me, but she did not move her head. I was really concerned about this mysterious problem with her neck, and though the nurses had gotten her a new wheelchair, they had merely put her in one with a higher back, neglecting to find and attach the neck and head support.

When I got Mom to the conference room, I sat with her hands in mine. I reminded her of the conversation we'd had a few days earlier about a move to Traverse City. I reminded her about the guardianship. She nodded that she understood. I asked the social worker and the notary public to come into the room.

When the social worker gave Mom a pen and she tried to get her hand to the table, I could not believe how much her hand was shaking. She'd never had tremors like this with her Parkinson's disease.

I took her hand, rested it on the edge of the table, and put the paper where she could sign it. I asked her to just make an X on the paper. The pen was a ballpoint and she could not put enough pressure on it to make it write. Finally, the social worker produced a felt-tipped pen. With the softer point, Mom was able to make a mark on the paper. It was a squiggly mark, not an "X." I was deeply alarmed and shocked at her inability to control the pen. How could her physical condition have declined so in just two weeks?

Glen came in and the nursing home employee and notary public left. We tried again to play cards, but Mom kept dropping hers on the floor. I had to help her play, as she seemed to have trouble distinguishing one suit from another. Then I gave her a mint. Mom had always liked the mints they have in certain restaurants, so I'd stopped at a restaurant supply store to buy some for her. I was dismayed to see the blue color from the coating on the candy drooling out of the right corner of her mouth. Of course, I did not know then that drooling is another of the adverse side effects of the antipsychotic.

When Mom suggested we stop playing, I was relieved. I told her that we would be back in a few days to pick her up and take her to Traverse City. Suddenly, Mom began to tremble. It seemed that her whole upper body was shaking. I got up, put my arms around her, and held onto her. She stopped shaking in about three minutes.

I asked Glen if he would sit with Mom while I went and talked to the nurse. I described what had just happened and asked whether Mom had been checked for the possibility of stroke. She didn't think so. She'd ask the physician. "This is to be expected," I heard again. I asked whether she could think of any other reason for what appeared to be a seizure to me. She had no explanation.

Adverse Drug Reactions

As described in Chapter Three, medication errors occur with alarming frequency. In addition, the risk is high that your loved one will suffer from medication side effects—also called adverse drug reactions. Medication errors and side effects can have life-threatening consequences.

Although federal laws are intended to protect the frail elderly in nursing homes from inappropriate drug use, your loved one cannot be guaranteed medical safety. The three primary reasons are the lack of training of health care professionals, the frequency with which inappropriate and dangerous medications continue to be used in U.S. nursing homes, and the limited time that nurses and doctors spend with nursing home residents. The cumulative result is that side effects are usually not adequately monitored.

As an important member of your loved one's team of caregivers, you need to learn how to evaluate medications, how to recognize medication errors and side effects, and to realize that you can help prevent adverse drug reactions. Changes in your loved one's status can alert you to the possibility that one or more of her medications is causing a problem. As I will continue to repeat, you don't need to be a doctor or nurse to recognize that something is wrong. You should always be aware of the potential for drug interactions and should always suspect a drug-drug, drug-disease, or drug-food interaction as the cause of a patient's symptoms.[1]

WHAT IS AN ADVERSE DRUG REACTION?

An "adverse drug reaction" (ADR) is an undesirable or unexpected event in response to a drug that requires a physician to alter the care of a patient. The physician may need to discontinue a drug, modify a dosage, prolong hospitalization, or administer supportive treatment. ADRs do not include drug withdrawal, drug-abuse syndromes, accidental poisonings, or complications of drug overdose.[2] Because it's common for the elderly to take many drugs, both prescription medications and over-the-counter drugs, it's no wonder that ADRs are common and pose a significant risk for elders.

The majority of drug-induced disorders result from drug-drug, drug-food, or drug-disease interactions. If your loved one suffers from an ADR, death is not necessarily the outcome. Instead, her quality of life may be decreased by damage to her mind's and body's ability to function normally, resulting in memory impairment, drowsiness, loss of coordination, confusion, and other symptoms.[3]

Some common ADRS include the following:

Urinary or bowel incontinence. These are a frequent side effect of medications. Since both problems cause embarrassing moments for your loved one, it's no wonder that she may try to cover up her difficulties, frustrating you and prolonging solutions. If you know that these annoying problems can be caused by medication side effects, you can avoid the anger and aggravation you might otherwise feel. Once you alert her physician to the problem and it is resolved by modifying her medications, everyone's life is easier and happier.

Sedation or dizziness. Many medications affect both logical thinking (cognition) and behavior. Some produce a state of apathy and inhibit initiative and emotions, and some can make your loved one drowsy or dizzy. These side effects are common and occur frequently. As you will learn in later chapters, they result in falls, dehydration, and protein/energy malnutrition.

Difficulty in swallowing or talking. Other side effects, often over-looked, are difficulties in swallowing and the ability to talk. If your loved one's swallowing is impaired, she will have trouble swallowing her medications. Or, as you will learn in Chapters Six and Seven, dehydration and protein/energy malnutrition may be fatal consequences. If her ability to talk is blocked, seek evaluation immediately. Treatment issues become even more difficult when your loved one is unable to communicate effectively with you, with her physician, and with other caregivers. As a result, her treatment will be compromised.

Bleeding. Many drugs cause bleeding, and some drugs like Coumadin and warfarin, which are used to prevent blood clotting, can lead to life-threatening bleeding episodes or anemia if taken with aspirin. Even over-the-counter pain relievers, if used improperly, can cause your loved one to have life-threatening bleeding episodes. This is particularly true if she suffers a silent gastrointestinal bleed. Unless detection is early and intervention is swift, she will likely die.

Tremor or rigidity. It is important that you, as a caregiver, understand the sudden onset of tremor as another "fire alarm." Tremor may indicate an adverse drug reaction, signaling neurological complications affecting the extrapyramidal system.[4] Tremor also occurs in PD patients whose Parkinson's medications need to be adjusted. Further, tremors can occur in patients who are suffering kidney failure whose regular prescription medications are not being properly eliminated by the kidneys so that drug levels accumulate to a toxic level. Extra-pyramidal symptoms cause involuntary motor movements such as tremor and/or abnormalities of muscle tone such as rigidity. These symptoms resemble the abnormal movements seen in patients with Parkinson's and are called "parkinsonism." Let me explain how these can be life- threatening to your loved one.

If your loved one suffers from Parkinson's disease (PD) and experiences a sudden worsening of tremor or rigidity, it is imperative that you alert her doctor to these symptoms. Ask whether the tremors may be considered as ADRs and may be reversible. Don't automatically assume, and encourage her physicians and nurses not to assume, that the sudden worsening of tremors are the normal progression of the disease. If you're wrong and her physician is wrong, the end result is that the ADR goes undetected, the drug is not withdrawn, and your loved one's health declines.

On the other hand, perhaps your loved one has not been diagnosed with PD. It is very common for an antipsychotic to interact with *undiagnosed* PD, resulting in an increase in tremor that is then diagnosed as PD. According to Dr. Friedman, there is a lag of weeks between the time an antipsychotic is prescribed and the cumulative effect of the blocking of dopamine caused by the drug. Eventually, so little dopamine is available to the basal ganglia that tremors are quite pronounced. But if the tremors that ensue are diagnosed as PD and the antipsychotic is not understood to be a causative factor, the drug may be continued, resulting in harm to the patient.

ADRS CAUSED BY ANTIPSYCHOTIC MEDICATIONS OFTEN PRESCRIBED IN THE ELDERLY

The most common side effects of typical antipsychotic medications are extrapyramidal side effects (EPSs). Between 50 and 75% of all patients taking antipsychotics experience EPSs.[5] Even medications prescribed for Parkinson's patients will cause EPSs if the dosage is incorrect or if something else, like dehydration or kidney failure, changes your loved one's ability to eliminate these drugs.

You will want to monitor your loved one to see if she develops EPSs. The most common of the acute EPSs are drug-induced parkinsonism, akinesia (lack of or slowed movement or expressionless face), dystonia (muscle rigidity and soreness), and akathisia (restlessness).

Dr. Kidder describes parkinsonism as involving such symptoms as slowed movement, depressed affect, drooling, tremor, and shuffling gait.[6] Document your observations. If your loved one, after taking a psychotropic drug, exhibits gait disorders, drooling, or tremor in excess of what was normal for her, you should be alarmed. You will want to call these changes to the attention of her nurses and physician. Elimination of drugs that block dopamine will usually resolve such problems.

Dystonia is another common drug-induced disorder. An acute dystonia involves muscle rigidity, contracted neck and eye muscles, and complaints of jaw and muscle soreness; it is frequently very painful. Neuroleptic medications such as antipsychotics can cause an acute dystonic reaction from a single dosage or tardive dystonia from chronic usage.[7]

How can you recognize a dystonia? In some patients, this means the neck is rigidly and painfully twisted, an effect over which the patient has no control. Such a patient is observed with her head lying at a painful-looking and distorted angle on her shoulder. A dystonia may also affect her ability to swallow and this will make drinking, eating, and talking very difficult, particularly when coupled with dysphagia (difficulty in swallowing caused by many medications).[8] Although a well-trained psychiatric nurse will usually identify a dystonia, you will want to make sure it is recognized and that appropriate treatment—usually elimination of the medication causing the condition—is undertaken. Some nurses, particularly in long-term care facilities, may not be as familiar with EPSs as are nurses who have regularly cared for psychiatric patients.

Another common EPS is akathisia, which involves pacing and restlessness or extremely uncomfortable subjective perceptions in which patients feel jumpy and unable to sit still or to concentrate.[9] A patient suffering from akathisia may appear to pick something (nothing) out of the air on a constant basis.

Even when an antipsychotic is used at low doses for short periods of time, from 30 to 50% of elderly patients may develop the EPS called tardive dyskinesia (TD).[10] TD causes varying symptoms such as a combination of abnormal involuntary muscle movements affecting the face, eyes, mouth, tongue, and limbs. TD can be very embarrassing to patients. Marked repetitive blinking can interfere with vision. In severe cases TD can be life-threatening, as when it affects the throat muscles and seriously interferes with breathing and swallowing.[11] TD is the most serious drug-induced EPS because it often lasts for months or years and can be irreversible even after the antipsychotic causing it is discontinued, especially in geriatric patients. In addition, although some interventions may help, there is no guaranteed treatment for it.[12] In younger patients, TD usually does not develop until one to two years or more of antipsychotic medication use, but the elderly are far more at risk for TD.[13]

Medical authorities recommend discontinuance of the responsible drug as the accepted response to the appearance of these side effects. Sometimes this helps, especially in the case of tremors and dystonia, but this assumes that the physician or staff has first detected that an adverse side effect has resulted from a medication.

COMMON DRUG-DRUG, DRUG-DISEASE, AND DRUG-FOOD INTERACTIONS

As discussed in Chapter Three, drug-drug interactions occur when side effects of one drug duplicate or intensify the side effects of another drug or, alternatively, counteract the intended beneficial action of another drug.

Many potential drug-drug interactions occur with the medications commonly prescribed for the elderly as well as with over-the-counter medications. See Appendix G for a list of interactions common to elderly patients.

Drug-disease interactions occur when a drug intensifies the physical or neurological symptoms of a patient's chronic disease or when, as a result of a chronic disease, the drug's intended action is increased or decreased. One common drug-disease interaction in the elderly occurs when a normal dosage of a medication that is eliminated through the kidneys interacts with impaired kidney function. For example, more than 90% of amantadine, a drug commonly prescribed for Parkinson's disease patients, is eliminated renally as unchanged drug. If kidneys are not functioning properly, amantadine is likely to accumulate, and seizures can occur.[14]

Cancer patients and survivors have their own set of complications. According to Dr. Wendy Harpham, an internist and long-term survivor of non-Hodgkin's lymphoma, cancer survivors who have been successfully treated with chemotherapy are especially at risk when treated for other ailments with drugs that are nephrotoxic—drugs that can cause kidney damage. Nephrotoxic drugs in doses that are considered normal for patients with the same characteristics such as age and weight can cause life-threatening kidney damage for those with a history of chemotherapy because that chemotherapy has caused subclinical damage to their kidneys.

So many complications can overlap that it is not unusual for body systems to be overwhelmed in the process. Imagine the cumulative effects of such conditions as dysphagia, dystonia, and parkinsonism—common side effects of drugs—when suffered by a frail elder with impaired kidney function. As these complications occur, drinking fluids becomes more difficult and patients may purposefully restrict fluids to avoid having to make it to the toilet in time to avoid an accident. It's easy to see how the cumulative effect of drugs and a decreased fluid intake can worsen kidney function, leading to dehydration, malnutrition, and drug toxicity.

Finally, drug-food interactions occur when food alters the way in which a drug acts in the body, either by intensifying the effects of the drug or by reducing or blocking the effects of the drug.

There are many common drug-food interactions, such as that which occurs between calcium and certain antibiotics that are commonly used in the elderly patient, including Levaquin, Cipro, and Bactrim DS.

Specifically, calcium blocks the absorption of antibiotics, reducing their effectiveness. These antibiotics should be taken two hours after and four hours before a patient eats any foods containing calcium such as milk, butter, cheese, and other milk products.

Another common drug-food interaction can occur when calcium is taken with thyroid medications, making the thyroid medication ineffective. An inverse kind of reaction is caused when calcium is taken with a diuretic used to eliminate excess water from the body (to treat edema). If thiazide diuretics are taken together with calcium, a dangerously high calcium level will result, which can lead to kidney failure.

Grapefruit juice is another food that commonly interacts with many medications. Whole grapefruit is also thought to cause an interaction. Grapefruit juice affects the metabolism of some drugs and as a result a greater dose of medication may be available in the bloodstream. With certain medications and in certain patients, the interaction can be fatal.

Common medications that are frequently taken by the elderly and that are known to interact with grapefruit juice include calcium channel blockers prescribed for heart problems and the treatment of blood pressure, statin drugs prescribed to lower cholesterol, certain antianxiety medications, certain antidepressants, certain bronchodilators, some antihistamines, and the men's impotency drug Viagra. For a more complete list of medications that should not be combined with grapefruit juice, see the Mayo Clinic's article "Is Grapefruit Juice Harmful? Hot Topics in Healthcare" at www.ahcpub.com/ahc_root_html/hot/archive/ima01152001.html.

Who Is Most at Risk?

If you are aware of what factors make patients at risk for ADRs, you will be in a better position to detect and prevent ADRs in your loved one. Dr. Beers and his colleagues identified the characteristics of those patients most likely to suffer an adverse drug reaction:

- Those who are elderly (more than 85 years of age)
- Those with decreased kidney function (less than 50 ml/min)
- Those who have more than six active chronic medical diagnoses
- Those taking more than 12 doses of several medications per day
- Those taking nine or more different medications per day (including over-the-counter and "as needed" or PRN medications)
- Those who have had a prior adverse drug reaction
- Those with low body weight or body mass index (<22 kg/m2)

Obviously, some persons will have more than one of these risk factors. Others may have all of them. These persons will be at a far greater risk of suffering an ADR.

Another reason why the elderly are more at risk for ADRS is that they take certain medications known to commonly result in ADRs. In Dr. Cooper's 1999 study, two classes of drugs were the predominant causes of the hospitalizations in elderly patients: NSAIDs, non-steroidal anti-inflammatory drugs typically used for arthritis that can cause gastrointestinal bleeding episodes that can be fatal, and psychotropic drugs, which are frequently implicated in falls with fracture.[15] Together, NSAIDs and psychotropic drugs accounted for 44 out of 64 hospitalizations in the elderly population.[16]

ADRS FOLLOWING HOSPITALIZATIONS

You'll need to be especially watchful for ADRs during your loved one's transition from hospital care to home. In February 2003, a report in the Annals of Internal Medicine revealed that nearly one in five people suffered an adverse medical event during the transition from hospital to home.[17] These ADRs were predominantly a result of being misdiagnosed or prescribed the wrong medication. Drug reactions causing rashes, constipation, and insomnia were the most common problem. The drugs most often causing the ADRs were as follows:

- Antibiotics (38% of patients)
- Corticosteroids (16%)
- Cardiovascular drugs (14%)
- Analgesics (including opiates) (10%)
- Anticoagulants (8%)

Of the patients affected, 11% went to an emergency department and 24% were readmitted to the hospital.

The researchers found that *one-third of the adverse events were preventable*. Another third were ameliorable—although they were unavoidable, their severity could have been decreased by earlier corrective action, according to this report.

Poor communication between the hospital caregivers, patients (and/or their family caregivers), and primary care physicians was cited as the most common reason why these ADRs occur. The report recommended that hospitals do more than simply send an email to a patient's primary care physician at the time of discharge detailing the new medication regimen.

The researchers recommended that hospitals specify exactly what these physicians need to do, when they should do it, and what they should watch for. In addition, hospitals should provide the same information to patients.[18]

What does this tell us? First, recall that lack of continuity of care is a huge threat to your loved one's health. Hospital care may not necessarily be provided by your loved one's primary doctor. Patients and their caregivers need to expect careful evaluation at the time of discharge. They need to be taught about their new drug therapies, the side effects they should watch for, and what they should do if specific problems develop. Caregivers should expect and request follow- up visits with hospitalists (specialists who provide hospital care to inpatients and act as a liaison with the primary care physician) within a week of discharge or follow-up telephone contact with a clinical pharmacist within five days of discharge as an additional procedure.[19]

ADRS IN NURSING HOMES

The facts are appalling. Adverse drug reactions are common in nursing homes. In August of 2000, Doctors Gurwitz and Avorn (leading advocates against the use of inappropriate medications in the elderly) and their colleagues conducted a study that assessed how often medication errors occurred and how serious they were. Errors determined to be drug-related were then categorized as either an adverse drug event or a potential adverse drug event. (Potential adverse drug events were those that might have harmed a patient but did not, either because of chance or because they were detected.[20])

Then Gurwitz and Avorn rated the ADRs by severity: significant, serious, life-threatening, or fatal. Examples of significant events included falls without an associated fracture, hemorrhages not requiring transfusion or hospitalization, and oversedation. Serious events were those such as falls with fracture, hemorrhages requiring transfusion or hospitalization, and delirium. Finally, a determination was made as to whether the ADR was preventable.[21]

ADRS ARE PREVENTABLE

Gurwitz and his colleagues found that *more than half* (51%) of the ADRs were preventable, including 72% of the fatal, life-threatening, or serious ADRs. They concluded that 34% of the significant ADRs were preventable. The errors were not commonly found in the areas of transcription, dispensing, or administration of the drugs. The most common errors were in choice of drug and monitoring of the drugs.[22]

Two categories of medications most often caused the preventable ADRs: psychoactive drugs[23] or anticoagulants. The most common types of preventable ADRs were neuropsychiatric events, including *delirium, dysphagia, and tremors*. The authors concluded that in order to prevent drug errors, physicians' attention should focus on the ordering (choosing the correct drug and dosage) and monitoring of drugs.

In August 2002, Dr. Gurwitz reported that "There may be as many as 20,000 fatal or life-threatening adverse drug events per year among the nursing home population; of these, 80% may be preventable."[24]

Elderly living in their own homes or family caregivers' homes are similarly at great risk for medication errors. In March 2003, Dr. Gurwitz and his colleagues published a review study involving a large group of Medicare enrollees. They found that elderly patients residing at home cared for by family physicians suffer significant numbers of ADRs, most of which may be preventable.[25] More than a quarter of the 1,523 ADRs were considered preventable (27.6%). Gurwitz found that the more serious the adverse drug reaction, the more likely it was thought to be preventable.

WHAT DRUGS SHOULD MAKE YOU SUSPICIOUS?

As a caregiver, you need to be alert to which drugs are known to cause the most frequent and preventable ADRS so that you can take a look at your loved one's drug regimen to assess the kind of risk to which she may be exposed.

In 1991, Dr. Beers[26] and his colleagues identified the factors that made elderly patients most at risk for adverse drug events, identified particular drugs and classes of drugs that are potentially dangerous and/or inappropriate for use in the elderly, and identified criteria to be used in prescribing for the elderly.[27] In 1997 and again in 2004, Dr. Beers, in collaboration with a panel of experts, updated and expanded upon this report.[28] Dr. Beers' research forms the basis for government regulations designed to protect the elderly from inappropriate and unnecessary drugs.

Certain drugs were identified by Beers as potentially dangerous for the elderly: Digoxin (used to treat arrhythmia), warfarin (a blood thinner, used to treat some heart disease), lithium (used to treat bi-polar disease), and chloropramide (used to treat diabetes or high blood sugar). Certain classes of medications identified as potentially dangerous included anticonvulsants, antipsychotics, benzodiazepines (both long-acting and intermediate-acting), narcotic analgesics, and anticholinergics.

The most common types of medications associated with preventable ADRs in Dr. Gurwitz's study in community-dwelling patients were:[29]

- Cardiovascular medications (24.5%)
- Diuretics (22.1%)
- Non-opioid analgesics (15.4%)
- Hypoglycemics (10.9%)

Dr. Gurwitz cited the following as the most common types of preventable ADRs:

- Electrolyte/kidney (26.6%)
- Gastrointestinal tract (21.1%)
- Excessive bleeding (15.9%)
- Metabolic/endocrine (13.8%)
- Neuropsychiatric events (8.6%)

What Can You Do to Help Detect and Manage Adverse Drug Reactions?

Effective management of patients to avoid, detect, and treat ADRs begins with knowing which patients are most at risk. Thus, you and your loved one's physician will consider the individual characteristics listed above to determine her risk for ADRs. As with the detection of delirium, the first clue that she's suffering an ADR will be some change in either her mental or physical status. If you know your loved one has several of the risk factors for ADRs that are listed above, you will be naturally suspicious whenever you see a change in status that could indicate she is experiencing an ADR. The more quickly an ADR is detected and the medication that is the culprit is reduced or eliminated, the greater the chance that she will avoid serious consequences. Then when a new medication is prescribed for your loved one, you should monitor her progress closely and alert her caregivers to signs of adverse reactions.

You must pay close attention to all drugs prescribed for your loved one. After all, who better than you? You know your loved one and her history, habits, interests, and social and emotional needs better than any staff person ever will. If a drug is causing a harmful condition in an elderly patient or exacerbating an existing condition, the person most likely to detect this is someone who observes the resident regularly and can appreciate any changes in status, someone who is suspicious enough to consider a medication as the cause, and someone who will be committed to finding a solution.

BACK UP YOUR SUSPICIONS

If you can openly communicate with your loved one's physician and nurses, the likelihood of averting harm is great, but you will also need to back up your suspicions with facts. In order to help your loved one avoid potential adverse drug reactions, you will need to:

Establish a Baseline for Your Loved One's Health. Acquire a three-ring binder and record your personal assessment of your loved one's mental, medical, and physical status on a regular basis, at least weekly. Include in your three-ring binder reproductions of the various appendices that are designed to help you and the staff assess her medical status. Update these checklists regularly, using the results of lab tests as they become available, to help you stay aware of your loved one's current status. This puts you in a position to help detect delirium, drug interactions, dehydration, malnutrition, and the other conditions discussed in this book.

It is crucial to write down your observations so that you have more to rely on than your memory should you need to advocate for a formal assessment by your loved one's physician or other caregivers or to alert them to the potential for a life-threatening situation. Use the form for making a history you will find in Appendix H. The facts you will accumulate in this history will help you to back up your suspicions that an ADR has occurred should you have to convince your loved one's physician. You can use the information in Appendix J to help you determine the degree of risk for ADRs that she has. Your written record of your loved one's medical, mental, and physical history will prove invaluable as you advocate for her.

Learn All You Can About Your Loved One's Disease(s). Because of the potential for drug-disease interactions, you will want to ask your loved one's physician whether a particular disease has any particular degenerative characteristics. Also ask whether any particular drugs or classes of drugs used to treat her disease interact with others in her drug regimen.

Keep a Record of All Medications Prescribed. It's important that you keep a record of all drugs your loved one is taking so that her physician may, if necessary, help determine potential ADRs. You can get package inserts for each medication prescribed for your loved one, including over-the-counter and "as needed" (PRN) drugs. If these are not made available to you by her physician, get them yourself. Most drug stores have package inserts, and package inserts for the top 200 prescription medications are available over the Internet.[30] If you don't have Internet access, your local library can access this website and print inserts for you or can give you copies of the information for each medication from the Physician's Desk Reference in the reference room. The information there is comparable to the package insert. Are there any specific warnings and/or contraindications in the package inserts associated with any drug that are related to your loved one's existing illnesses and/or existing drug regimen? If so, tell her physician.

Keep track of which medications are introduced, eliminated, increased, or reduced in dosage. You can use Appendix I to create a record for her medications and to keep track of any side effects she might suffer.

Advocate for a Reduction in Medications. The best way to protect your loved one is to see that she is as free from medications as possible. Therefore, when you have learned about her diseases and conditions and the medications prescribed for them, you should be in a position to advocate for changes or reductions in medications as appropriate. Remember that the more medications an elderly person takes, the greater the risk of harm. Look for opportunities to help free your loved one from unnecessary medications. Advocate with her physicians to consider changes in her drug regimen to medications that may be safer, or to consider a reduction in dosages where possible, particularly if her lab tests show that her kidneys have decreased function.

Ask About Alternatives to NSAIDs. Because NSAIDs are so dangerous for the elderly, you will want to avoid them if possible. One way is to use medication administered through the skin instead of the gut. The following painkillers are available in varying strengths as a sustained-release medication administered through a transdermal patch: fentanyl, oxycodone, methadone, and morphine. Be aware that these are usually prescribed for extreme pain such as that suffered by cancer patients.

Another compound people frequently use to reduce arthritis pain is SAM-e (S-Adenosyl-Methionine), pronounced "Sammy." Although

SAM-e has been available as a prescription drug in Europe for twenty years, it was only introduced in the United States in February 1999.

In recent years, glucosamine and chondroitin have been widely promoted as a treatment for osteoarthritis. These are thought to relieve arthritis pain and stiffness and have fewer side effects than NSAIDs. They are also thought to promote the formation and repair of cartilage, to promote water retention and elasticity in joints, and to inhibit the enzymes that break down cartilage. While these claims have not been supported by much in the way of reliable research, my orthopeaedic surgeon not only recommends them, he uses them himself. But he laughs as he says: "Americans have the most expensive urine in the world," referring to how we eliminate the many vitamins, supplements, and medications Americans take in every day. As with any medication, it is best to consult with your loved one's physician before starting to take any supplements such as SAM-e, glucosamine, and/or chondroitin.

Prevention of ADRs: Safe Medication Use

DRUG SAFETY IN THE HOSPITAL

If your loved one is admitted to a hospital, you will want to do the following:

Perform a complete drug review. Take with you a complete list of all medications your loved one is taking. Better yet, take all of the medications so there is no mistake about dosages. Be sure to include all prescription and over-the-counter drugs, herbal products, and other supplements. Now her physician will know exactly what she's been taking.

Find out about her medications. Ask the name and purpose of every drug your loved one is given. There are two goals intended here. First, you will be informed. Second, you will ensure that drugs are not administered by mistake.

Learn the correct dosage. Ask a professional to explain dosages to you. Optimally, you will ask her admitting primary care physician, but if she is not available, you should ask her nurse or the hospital staff.

Find out what it looks like. Know what her medicine looks like. Speak up right away if she's given something that looks different. Ask whether the brand or dosage was changed. Make sure there is no mistake.

Make sure they have the right patient. Make sure the staff checks her identification band before administering any medication.

Monitor new drugs. If your loved one is hospitalized, she probably doesn't feel very well. Be sure to monitor new drugs and alert her physician or the staff if you notice adverse side effects such as diarrhea, fever, tremor, headache, nausea, rash, etc.

Discuss medication thoroughly at discharge. At discharge, ask questions about any new medicines prescribed for your loved one. Be sure you and she know what each one is for, how it should be taken (for example with food or without food), what she should do if she misses a dose, what side effects she should watch for, and whether the drug interacts with any particular foods or herbs.

DRUG SAFETY AT THE PHYSICIAN'S OFFICE

Each time you take your loved one to see her physician you should again do a drug review. Take her medications to her office in a brown bag.

Learn about her medications. Be sure to ask her physician about all new drugs she prescribes. Take notes. Ask the physician these questions: What is the brand name? Is there a generic, and what is its name? What is the purpose of the drug? What is the dosage? Are there any special instructions about how to take it? How long is your loved one to take it? Does her physician have any other written information about the drug?

Do a complete drug review. Ask her physician if there are any medications that can be eliminated or reduced.

DRUG SAFETY AT THE PHARMACY

You can also help keep your loved one safe at the pharmacy by doing the following:

Consolidate all of her prescriptions at one pharmacy. Her pharmacist will be able to monitor for drug-drug interactions if all prescriptions are filled at the same pharmacy. Her pharmacist may even have a computer program that flags potentially dangerous drug combinations. This is particularly important when your loved one has several different physicians, each of whom may be prescribing medications, such as a cardiovascular physician to monitor heart disease, an internist as a primary care doctor, an endocrinologist to monitor diabetes, etc.

Talk to her pharmacist about her medications and get written information. The pharmacist may be able to give you package inserts. A patient information sheet describing everything you need to know about the drug is usually dispensed with every prescription, especially if this is a new drug for her. If you don't get one, ask for it. Then read it.

Disclose all medications, including over-the-counter ones. Be sure the pharmacist knows all the medicines your loved one takes, including herbal remedies and OTC meds. Too often elders forget that these medications may interact with their prescribed drugs.

Be sure to double-check all refills. When you refill prescriptions, if the packaging or the product looks different from the last one, ask why. Mix-ups don't often occur, but they do happen.

DRUG SAFETY AT HOME

Keep your loved one safe at home by following a few safety tips:

Know what she's taking. Leave drugs in their original containers. Always read the information sheet from the pharmacy before giving her any drug. Read the label each time you dispense it.

Observe special instructions. Some drugs must be taken with food, and others should be taken without. Some, such as the drugs dispensed to cure or treat bone loss, must be taken sitting up and the patient must remain sitting for at least one half hour. Some may be taken at the same time such as multiple vitamins and calcium supplements, but some drugs such as thyroid and some antibiotics interact with calcium and thus you will need to schedule the drugs either two to four hours before or two to four hours after her vitamins and calcium. Many drugs interact with grapefruit juice and other foods.

Establish a schedule for her medications. Make a written schedule for her medications and try to stick to it. Make sure she doesn't take more medicine or take it more often than she's told. Unless her physician directs otherwise, give her the medicine in the evening.

Check her daily intake. If she takes more than three prescription drugs, you should be sure to check her daily intake of medicines. Be sure she is on schedule. There are several types of medication organizers available. If your loved one lives at home and does not have 24-hour care, you may want to provide her with an organizer to ensure that she takes the right medication at the right time. One such organizer has little boxes for seven days. Each day is divided into four separate boxes. The cap for each has easy-to-read raised letters marked MORN, NOON, EVE. AND BED.

If you are concerned about whether she'll remember to take her medications on time, other medication trays have a built-in talking reminder that operates on AAA batteries. There are four programmable dosage-time settings and a missed-pill alert. The alarm can be set as a beeper, silent flashing light, or voice mode ("Time to take your pill.").

Keep a medication diary. Be sure to write down the names of medications she's taking and note any reactions to the drugs or symptoms she experiences such as rash, headache, stomachache, nausea, tiredness, confusion, constipation, etc.

What happens if she misses a dose? Find out what to do if she misses a dose or forgets to take her medication. If this happens, usually she should take it as soon as she can, but if it is almost time for her next dose, she should skip the missed dose and wait until the usual time to take the medicine. She usually should never double up to make up for a missed dose.

Be sure the drug is finished. To ensure optimal drug therapy, be sure your loved one takes the medication until it is gone. Don't stop using the medication when her symptoms end.

Throw away old drugs. Discard all expired drugs, unless her doctor or pharmacist says that they can be safely used.

Get rid of drugs she doesn't need. Discard drugs her physician says she should no longer take.

Be sure she can see the drug labels. Your loved one shouldn't take drugs in darkness or without her reading glasses, even if she is sure she's grabbing the right bottle.

Be alert to signs of drug side effects. Call your loved one's physician right away if she has any of these side effects:

- Muscle pain, weakness, or cramps
- Red-purple rash on her nose or cheeks, swelling around her eyes
- Skin rash or hives
- Stomach pain, nausea, vomiting, loss of appetite
- Unexplained fever
- Yellow skin or eyes

If she has problems with these less serious side effects, tell her doctor:

- Constipation or diarrhea
- Headache
- Mild stomach upset, gas, indigestion

Avoid drug mishaps. Store all medicines including OTCs well out of reach of children.

I urge you not to be lulled into a sense of security as I was. These medical issues are very complex. Whether your loved one lives at home or in a nursing facility, you are undoubtedly spending far more time with her than her medical caregivers and your observations can be very helpful to her physicians. If you are knowledgeable and vigilant, you can give her an added level of protection from common adverse drug reactions.

CHAPTER FIVE

Falls: A Significant Cause of Harm to the Elderly

OCTOBER 2000

Mom had fallen several times in September. The most serious fall was on Sep-tember 17, when she broke several ribs and severely bruised her face. Because my sisters and I were unaware that the falls were not "accidents" but were signs of serious medical and medication issues, we were not alarmed by these falls. We were concerned, of course. We were sad about her decline. But the nurses assured us that what was occurring was normal, was expected, and that there was nothing that could be done.

After Mom's transfer from the skilled nursing unit to the extended care unit on October 13, 2000, the nurses' notes frequently documented her "confusion," her chronic constipation, her known metabolic disorder, her lack of balance, and her continuing falls. In fact, in the extended care unit, Mom was confined to a wheelchair. An alarm was attached between her wheelchair and her clothing to alert the nursing staff if she tried to stand unassisted.

Mom's records show that she fell twice more in late October. The nurses found her on the floor. Mom had previously been scolded for trying to get up without assistance. She was, I am sure, worried about being scolded and did not want to admit she was "at fault." When Mom was helped off the floor on one of these occasions she told the nurse, "I didn't fall. I was supposed to be down here." The nurse noted in her records that the "fall is not due to medications." Unfortunately, the antipsychotic Mom was being given and her worsening elec-trolyte imbalance causing delirium were not considered as causes for these falls. Thus, there was no intervention.

Falls: A Common Occurrence

You should never think of falls as "accidents," or think they are unpredictable and unavoidable. In fact, medical research has identified falls as common, frequent, predictable, and often preventable occurrences in the elderly.

Think of falls the same way you do delirium—as a "fire alarm." Recognize that falls may have a direct, detrimental, and sometimes deadly impact on your loved one's life expectancy and quality of life. Studies show that a significant number of the elderly who fall die within a year of a fall. Also recognize that falls are an important clue that there is something wrong with your loved one that should be investigated immediately. Often you will find that a new disease process or condition needs to be treated or a medication needs to be discontinued, changed, or reduced. Like delirium, falls often signify an underlying medical disease or condition that, if undetected and untreated, may lead to death.

Falls Can Be Deadly

Studies show that a significant number of the elderly who fall die within a year of a fall.

INCIDENCE AND CONSEQUENCES OF FALLS

Consider how falls can compromise your loved one's quality of life in light of the following facts:

- one-sixth of all deaths in persons over 65 years of age are caused by accidents, and two-thirds of those deaths are caused by falls;
- 40% of traumatic injuries occurring in the elderly population are caused by falls.[1]

The older your loved one is, the more susceptible she is to falling. Every year, one-third of persons over the age of 65 living in their own homes or the homes of family caregivers fall. Half of those over 80 years of age living independently fall. Those elderly who are hospitalized or live in nursing homes fall far more frequently than those living in the community. Up to half of those living in nursing homes fall each year; more than 40% of them fall more than once each year. Some researchers believe that even these dramatic statistics underestimate the rate of falls, many of which may be unreported.[2]

Falls can be deadly. About 10,000 elderly persons die every year in the U.S. as a result of injuries suffered in falls. Over one-third of these deaths occur among persons older than 85 years. The vast majority of these deaths are related to hip fractures; patients with hip fractures are 15 to 20 times more likely to die than those who have not had a fracture.[3] Even when falls do not cause death, they can cause significant disability in the elderly, such as minor soft tissue injuries, hip fractures, other types of fractures, and serious soft tissue injuries.[4]

Death or physical injuries caused by falls are not the only serious consequence for the elderly. An elderly person who has fallen is three times more likely to be placed in a nursing home than an elderly person who has not fallen. Up to two-thirds of those who survive a hip fracture lose and do not regain bodily function.

Consider, too, that falls also pose a serious threat to your loved one's psychological and physical health, or both. Her fear of falling may cause social isolation and depression when she restricts prior activities such as church attendance, travel, and shopping. Fear of falling may even cause her to avoid such normal activities of daily living as bathing or getting dressed.[5] She might restrict fluid intake so she doesn't have to rush to the bathroom, risking another fall. Dehydration and kidney failure might result. Because of the serious consequences falls can have, it is important to figure out what is causing them so that you can help to prevent future falls.

What Causes Falls?

When your loved one falls, you will need to figure out the reason or reasons before you can figure out how to prevent future falls. Don't assume there is only one cause. In fact, there may be several reasons why she fell. Extrinsic factors contributing to falls include environmental hazards as well as activity-related factors. Intrinsic factors contributing to falls are characteristics that are inherent to your loved one related to aging, disease, or medication.

EXTRINSIC FACTORS

Extrinsic factors, also called environmental factors, play an important role in the elderly person's falls. In most studies, 50% of falls deemed to be "accidents" are related to some environmental cause.

To help detect the cause of a fall and help prevent your loved one from falling in the future, carefully evaluate her home to find and eliminate environmental hazards. Does her home have loose rugs, slippery floors, and uneven door thresholds? [6] Does she have stacks of books and newspapers on the floor that she could trip over? Have you looked at her bathroom fixtures and home furnishings? These can commonly cause falls. Are her fixtures inappropriately low or high? Do they lack arm supports or rails? Stairs account for about 10% of falls. How do hers measure up? Does she have adequate handrails? Does she need a safer step-stool in the kitchen in order to reach things in upper cupboards? What about her vision? Both loss of vision acuity and weakness in the lower extremities may cause her to fall on stairs. Are there areas in her home where poor lighting compounds her failing visual acuity? You will undoubtedly find many environmental traps that are just "an accident waiting to happen."

INTRINSIC FACTORS

Intrinsic factors are your loved one's unique characteristics that may be a second reason why she fell and is at risk to fall in the future. These factors account for the remaining 50% of falls the elderly suffer. The intrinsic factor that most often causes falls is a lack of balance. This may be due to a physical or medical condition or may relate to side effects from a medication.

Aging Contributes to Falls

According to Dr. Kenneth Steinweg, diseases and age-related changes contribute to falls or "accidents" often blamed on environmental factors. Persons 75 or younger are more likely to fall because of environmental causes. Multiple medical conditions and the concomitant use of many medications to treat them are more likely to be the cause of falls in those over the age of 85.

Unfortunately, many factors impair the key organ systems involving balance.[7] Maintaining a stable, upright position is a complex process involving a number of systems. To stay balanced, one's brain must work together with musculoskeletal coordination; moreover, other body systems need to function well, too. If your loved one is dizzy or light-headed or if her breathing is labored, she is at a greater risk of falling. Illnesses or conditions and the medications she takes to treat them can all impair her balance. Often, more than one of these factors is involved. You can work together with your loved one's physician to figure out which of these is affecting her balance and causing her to fall.

Patient Characteristics That Contribute to Falls

Dizziness, lightheadedness
Impaired consciousness, delirium
Bowel and bladder problems
Age-related factors
Vision problems
Chronic illnesses
Medical conditions

There are many other age-related physiologic factors, common to the elderly, that impact your loved one's alertness, balance, and mobility in various ways. For example, aging frequently results in gait changes. This in turn affects balance, which contributes to a predisposition to fall.

If your loved one has not done much weight-bearing activity, this will also affect her balance, as her muscles will have atrophied as a result. For that reason, you'll want to be proactive in dealing with your loved one if she falls and then reacts by becoming sedentary because she fears falling again. If her fears are not dealt with, this sedentary lifestyle will, in fact, increase her risk of falling.

CHRONIC CONDITIONS AND ILLNESSES

Many acute and chronic conditions and illnesses (i.e., urinary tract infections, pneumonia, myocardial infarctions, arrhythmias, and so on) make the elderly more at risk for falls. Thus, falling can be a "red alert" in the same way that delirium can be so that caregivers begin to look for a previously undetected medical disease or condition that should be treated.

Your loved one's situation may be complicated because she has numerous risk factors for falls—has several chronic conditions and also takes several medications per day. If, for example, she takes five or more medications per day, has had a stroke, and suffers from dysphagia, with dehydration and protein/energy malnutrition occurring as a result, she has a much greater risk of falling than an elderly person who has only one risk factor.

Is your loved one delirious? Altered consciousness will impair balance. It will affect what she sees or feels, how she reacts to what she sees or feels, and how her body is able to respond to what she sees or feels, all of which make her vulnerable to falls. Some of these diseases and/or the medications used to treat them will make your loved one feel dizzy, increasing the likelihood of falls. Bowel and bladder problems can also increase the risk of falls because they cause her to hurry to the bathroom. While those conditions that affect the lower extremities are most important, if she is chronically dehydrated or under-nourished, she has an increased risk for falls.

Your loved one may not see as well as she used to; lack of visual acuity plays an extremely important role in the loss of balance. Consider whether her ability to perceive contrasts and spatial detail has decreased as a normal part of the aging process. Other problems related to visual acuity causing falls common to the elderly are the ability to adapt to light and dark and also to accommodate to changes in distance. All of these factors may impact your loved one's balance.

Some of the other conditions commonly associated with a greater risk of falls are arthritis, stroke, dementia, Parkinson's disease, hip fractures, peripheral neuropathies, amputation, foot disorders and deformities, and orthostatic hypotension, which can be caused by heart disease and also many medications.

Additionally, electrolyte and metabolic imbalances, hypothyroidism, hypoglycemia, dehydration, malnutrition, diabetes, cardiac arrhythmias, valvular heart disease, syncope (fainting), and lumbar stenosis (a degenerative narrowing of the spinal canal, common in the elderly) will also make your loved one more likely to fall.

MEDICATIONS

Many medications also put the elderly at a greater risk for falls, and the greater the number of medications and dosages your loved one takes, the more her risk increases. Falling may be the signal that a medication should be discontinued, changed, or reduced.

The drugs most often cited as causing falls are sedatives, antianxiety medications, antidepressants, antihypertensives, and antipsychotics. Antihypertensives, which cause postural hypotension, are linked to 3 to 23%

of falls in the elderly.[8] Concommitant use of diuretics, anticholinergics, and the medications cited immediately above will also increase her risk.

Medications That Contribute to Falls

Sedatives
Antianxiety medications
Antidepressants
Antihypertensives
Antipsychotics

Antipsychotic medications may directly lead to falls because their side effects can make your loved one drowsy, dizzy, less acutely aware, and can impact her normal ability to react to a hazard (such as a change in the level of the floor crossing a threshold) and/or avoid it. Those patients receiving medications that are long-acting or those receiving three or more medications a day are most at risk. As the number of medications increases, the risk increases exponentially. The use of antipsychotic medications also doubles the risk of recurrent falls, even after controlling for dementia, depression, and other risk factors.[9]

Help Your Loved One's Doctor Detect the Specific Cause of Falls

Developing a plan to reduce your loved one's risk for falling is important in order to maintain her health and quality of life. The first step will be to properly assess her unique risk for falls. Nursing homes are required to do this, and they give some risk factors more weight than others because some are more likely to result in falls than others.

You can use Appendix K to assess your loved one's risk of falling. Keep a copy in your medical record and update it as necessary. To thoroughly evaluate her, you will also need to ferret out the details of any past falls to unearth important clues.

HISTORY

Start by taking your loved one's history. Witnesses to her falls may be able to provide valuable clues. Learning what happened immediately preceding a fall may likewise provide important clues. If your loved one was changing position just before a fall, symptoms of lightheadedness, suggestive of orthostatic hypotension, should be considered. An arrhythmia may be suggested by the presence of palpitations. Did she experience a loss of consciousness, incontinence, or confusion? Because the strongest predictor of falls is a previous fall, it is important to tell her physician whether there were prior falls. Recurrent falls are much more likely to result from intrinsic factors.

Because medications are a significant cause of falls, be suspicious. All medications taken, including "as needed" or PRN medications and over-the-counter drugs, should be reviewed with your loved one's physician. Those medications most often implicated as causing falls should be looked at skeptically.

Co-morbid conditions such as arthritis, a previous stroke, or cardiac conditions should be considered as causes for a fall as well. Thus, your loved one's past medical history often provides important clues to instability. Have your loved one's physician review her musculoskeletal and neurologic system since deficits there contribute to falls. Don't forget that inactivity may cause debilitation of the musculoskeletal system because of bone demineralization or loss of muscle strength, so let her physician know if she's become sedentary. Additionally, her physician may want to consider whether her inactivity has caused decreased cardiovascular and respiratory capacity and has decreased oxygen levels in her brain, making her dizzy and precipitating her falls.

PHYSICAL EXAMINATION

Your loved one's physician may perform a physical examination to identify intrinsic factors or to validate factors detected in her history. After she's fallen, her physician will pay special attention to the following:

Vital signs. To see if your loved one has developed orthostatic hypotension, her physician will check her blood pressure and pulse rate both while she is lying down and after she's been standing for five minutes. Because an acute illness can precipitate a fall, your loved one's temperature should be checked for a slight increase or decrease. An increased respiratory rate may be the only sign of congestive heart failure, pneumonia, or early sepsis (infection). Recent weight loss will signal dehydration or serious illness, both contributors to falls.

Mental status testing. Your loved one's physician will assess her mental status to help determine the cause of a fall. The medical journal I have urged you to keep will be invaluable here, particularly if the examining physician does not know your loved one. Your observations, backed up by your written (and historical) assessments of her mental status, may be essential to obtaining an accurate assessment.

While it is certainly true that a fall might make your loved one suddenly "loopy," it goes without saying that an abnormal mental status should never be accepted as a normal consequence of a fall. Instead, you'll want to advocate for further evaluation to determine whether your loved one is delirious or has suffered an injury to the brain. Failure to make an accurate determination may prove life-threatening to the patient, because if the confusion is attributed solely to the fall, an underlying disease process may go undetected and untreated, leading to her death.

Examination. Your loved one's physician should next make a thorough examination of her head and neck, cardiac, musculoskeletal, and neurologic systems, focusing on areas that are the most likely causes of falls. Testing of visual fields and hearing should be included. Range of motion and muscle strength should be assessed, including gait and balance testing. The feet should also be checked to see if any foot problems such as calluses, corns, or nail problems could have caused the fall.

Laboratory testing. Your loved one's history, including a chart review for recent laboratory data, the physical examination, and the gait and balance testing will determine what laboratory testing is appropriate. While there are no recommended tests to be performed in elderly persons who experience a fall, her physician will recommend testing to detect some of the common and complex medical problems frequently occurring in the elderly population that can contribute to falls. If her physician suspects a cardiac event, she will order an electrocardiogram. If a urinary tract infection or dehydration is suspected, urine or blood tests will be ordered. If a medical illness or condition is suspected as a cause of a fall, the generally recommended tests include a complete blood count, measurement of electrolytes, blood urea nitrogen and creatinine tests, and a urinalysis.

Because of your unique knowledge of your loved one's condition and environment, you are in the best position to help her physician identify the cause or causes of falls, as well as to help her prevent falls. Based upon my experiences with Mom, if your loved one lives in a nursing facility, I suggest you pay special attention to how the nursing home identifies the causes of falls and seeks to remedy them.

Intervention: Treatment and Elimination
of Causes of Falls

Understanding the contributing factors, treating medical conditions caus-ing falls, and reducing risk are the keys to prevention of falls. Your recog-nition of the intrinsic and extrinsic causes of falls as discussed above will help you and your loved one's medical caregivers identify specific strategies to reduce the likelihood of her falling again. Specific care plans to prevent future falls will involve one or more of the following: (a) treatment of acute or reversible physical or medical conditions (intrinsic factors) that are identified as a cause of her fall, (b) elimination of the environmental (extrinsic) factors that are identified as a cause of her fall, and (c) consid-eration and use of adaptive devices to counteract irreversible deficits.[10]

TREATMENT OF ACUTE OR
REVERSIBLE CONDITIONS THAT CAN BE
A CAUSE OF FALLS

A clear example of the first category, treating acute or reversible condi-tions, would be the treatment of a specific illness or condition known to be associated with falls such as pneumonia, congestive heart failure, or a urinary tract infection. Clearly, curing a disease or condition that makes your loved one weak, feverish, or dizzy will eliminate some risk of falls.

REDUCE OTHER CAUSES OF FALLS

The second category, reducing the cumulative burden of causative factors, includes improving your loved one's ability to see, improving footwear or providing foot care if needed, and eliminating or reducing medication dosages. In fact, one of the most modifiable risk factors is usually medica-tion use. To eliminate risks associated with medication use, you should use the "brown-bag" method of evaluating your loved one's medications with her doctor that was described in Chapter Four. Focus on these issues:

- Identifying specific medications associated with increased risk of falls (for example, psychotropic or cardiovascular medications)
- Recognizing recent changes in medications
- Assessing the potential to reduce the number of medications and/or the number of dosages taken each day

Another way you can greatly reduce the likelihood that your loved one will fall again is to encourage and facilitate her in weight-bearing exercises and strength training. You've heard the phrase "use it or lose it." Nowhere does this phrase apply with so much impact as here. If your loved one doesn't exercise to keep up her muscle tone and keep her joints limber, she will be very much at risk for falling. The more she neglects this area of her life and the longer she neglects it, the harder it will be for her to rebuild atrophied muscle mass, to get up and walk, and to walk without tottering and falling. Both agility and strength impact significantly on her ability to remain upright. Getting her out to walk, taking her to senior aerobics at a local pool, participating in a local tai chi group or other strength-building exercise program—all of these activities will help eliminate a huge potential for falls.

PROVIDE ADAPTIVE TOOLS TO IMPROVE SAFETY

The third way to intervene to reduce the risk of falls involves introducing safety devices to help protect your loved one if she is physically unstable. Canes, walkers, or protective rails in the home are some examples of adaptive tools. You might work with a physical therapist to determine which type of intervention is most appropriate for your loved one and will be most likely to reduce or eliminate what puts her at risk for falls in the first place.

OTHER PREVENTATIVE MEASURES

Some additional common-sense things can be done to lessen the potential for falls. Since most falls (75%) occur in the home, if your loved one remains at home you can reduce her risks by making the home environment safer:

1. Examine the lighting in the home. In particular, look for and eliminate dark shadows in doorways or on stairs. Install night-lights in hallways, the bedroom, and bathroom. Consider installing a "Clapper"—a device that turns a lamp on at the sound of a hand clap.
2. Inspect all rugs. Remove throw rugs, tack down loose ends, and/or use a non-skid backing.
3. Inspect the stairways and fix loose boards or carpet. Install handrails on both sides of the stairwell. Be sure stairways are well lit.

4. Inspect the home for clutter. Books and magazines should be up off the floor so your loved one doesn't trip over them. Cords for lamps or extension cords must be tucked away from trafficked areas or covered by flooring.
5. Install handrails in the bathroom to assist your loved one in using the bathtub, the shower, and the toilet.
6. Inspect the kitchen. Put frequently used items within easy reach, not too low and not too high. Try to make things accessible so that your loved one will not need a stepladder or high stool.

In a similar manner, you can lessen the potential for falls by preventing the conditions and diseases that can cause falls:

1. Make sure your loved one sees her eye doctor once a year or as needed to correct cataracts and other eye diseases.
2. Examine her feet. You may need to schedule an appointment with a foot doctor to take care of large, thick nails and corns, since most elderly people are unable to care for their own feet. Many communities have regular foot care clinics sponsored by senior centers or the Agency on Aging where low-cost foot care is available.
3. Look at her footwear. Shoes that lack support and/or have slippery soles account for many falls. Your loved one should wear shoes that provide traction for safety. Slippers are completely inappropriate and should be avoided.
4. Take a look at your loved one's medication list. Check your records to see which medications are associated with an increased risk of falls. Talk to her physician about these medications, about the side effects of the medications, and also about the number of medications. Accumulation of side effects is a heavy predictor of falls. If you can work with her physician to minimize the number of medications, you can eliminate some of the risk. Do any dosages need to be reduced in light of dehydration and reduced kidney function?
5. Ask your loved one about dizzy spells. If she has dizzy spells, consult with her physician to find out why.
6. Investigate whether bowel or bladder control issues are affecting the way in which your loved one moves. Rushing to the bathroom to avoid an "accident" is a reason behind many falls. While reinforcing the need for fluids in important, this encouragement needs to be balanced with concern for attention to safe

toileting methods. Encourage frequent trips to the bathroom to avoid additional risks for falling.

7. There are many products available to minimize the embarrassment of minor urinary incontinence ("dribbling") such as pads and padded briefs. Use of these products should be encouraged if concern about soiling clothing or rugs is a reason why your loved one hurries to the bathroom. If she's embarrassed using incontinence pads, remind her that many companies are spending millions of dollars on advertising programs on TV during peak hours for senior viewers. Obviously, she's not the only one with this problem. Some of these companies now offer "discreet home delivery." You can go to GOOGLE.COM to find a source for incontinence pads that will be delivered to her door.[11] A bedside commode might solve nighttime toileting concerns. Look to see whether the path from bed to toilet is clear and well lighted to avoid falls in the night.

8. Discuss with her physician whether physical therapy would help your loved one learn safer ways of getting up from a chair or the bed or safer ways of transferring from chair to bed. Sometimes, particularly after an elderly patient has been released from the hospital after treatment of injuries caused by falls, Medicare will pay for in-home physical therapy two to three times a week.

9. Consider whether your loved one can and should use the facilities of a nearby health club to do specific resistance exercises to strengthen and maintain muscles in her legs, ankles, feet, and back and to maintain balance. Remember, however, that during flu season, frail people vulnerable to infection should probably not use a public health club because of the prevalence of germs. Some hospitals maintain "healthy heart" facilities for the elderly that may present an alternative, safer option for exercise.

10. Encourage your loved one to use a cane or walker if she is unsteady when walking and if her physician suggests or approves it.

11. Consider attaching an alarm to your loved one's clothing and then to the wheelchair to alert caregivers if she tries to get up alone if your loved one is in a nursing home, has impaired mobility, is in a wheelchair, and/or has mental status changes that cause her to try to walk or stand unassisted.

12. Encourage your loved one to stand up slowly. When she awakens, encourage her to sit on the side of the bed a few minutes

before standing up to give her blood pressure time to adjust. If your loved one gets up too quickly, her blood pressure may be too low, causing her to be light-headed, to lose balance, and to fall. This brief orthostatic hypertension can be avoided with careful habits.

Whether your loved one resides in a nursing home, her own home, or your home, use an organized approach to discover the factors that put her at risk for falls, to get treatment of medical causes of falls, to make environmental changes in her home, and to institute use of adaptive tools such as a cane or walker in order to eliminate or lessen her risk. Everything you can do to improve her stability when walking will help to prevent falls. This, in turn, will add immeasurably to your loved one's longevity and quality of life.

CHAPTER SIX

Dehydration: Water, Water Everywhere and Not a Drop to Drink

NOVEMBER 4-5, 2000

Jill took Mom's sister, Leona, to see Mom before I transferred Mom to the new nursing home in Traverse City on November 6. When she and Leona arrived at Alpine Manor at about 11:00 a.m. on Saturday, November 4, Mom was in bed asleep. They were unable to wake her, so they decided to go out to lunch and come back later. When they came back at about 1:30 p.m., Mom was still in bed and asleep. They did not wake her.

The following day, Jill and Leona again went to see Mom at about 11:00 a.m. Once again, she was in bed asleep. They roused her and talked to her for a while and Mom seemed to recognize Leona at the end of the bed. The nurses told Jill that Mom had been in bed since Friday and that she had had nothing to eat or drink in all that time.

After Jill's call on November 5, I telephoned Alpine Manor and requested that they hydrate Mom because I was worried she would be too dehydrated to survive the trip. I did not know that Alpine Manor was not equipped for and had no staff trained or available to insert an IV for simple hydration. I was told that the nurse would check with a doctor and would call me back.

The medical records for that last weekend contain contradictory information. They show that the nurse I spoke with told me that Mom was eating and drinking 100% that was offered and fluids were being offered every hour. Her nursing notes also show that she told one of the staff doctors the same thing and also told him that Mom was alert and responsive. The doctor did not order hydration. The nurse later talked to Jill and was able to convince Jill that nothing needed to be done.

Notes in Mom's records written by other health care workers and a staff doctor show that Mom was "in bed sleeping" from Friday through Monday morning, that she was not responding to verbal or non-verbal cues, and that her lips were dry and cracked, a sign of dehydration. One nurse noted, "Staff report not taking fluids." In fact, a staff doctor was called to Mom's bedside twice during the weekend and it is obvious from his notes that he thought Mom was dying. This doctor diagnosed Mom with delirium and a "probable urinary tract infection." He ordered an antibiotic and discontinued the antipsychotic. He ordered lab tests for Monday. Neither he nor the facility notified me or my sisters that Mom's condition had changed for the worse.

On Sunday the doctor saw Mom again. He noted her electrolyte imbalance as a cause for her delirium. Unfortunately, his diagnosis of dehydration and delirium was not made a part of the discharge documents transmitted to the Traverse City nursing home. The lab test results from that day were not included either. As a result, when Mom arrived in Traverse City, her working diagnosis, in the words of the Alpine Manor medical director, was "general debilitation secondary to pelvic fracture." No one in Traverse City was expecting delirium, dehydration, or malnutrition.

—□—

Dehydration: The Most Common Fluid and Electrolyte Disorder

You may be surprised to learn that dehydration is epidemic among the elderly population, both in long-term care settings and in home-dwelling elders. Because it is difficult to detect in its early stages and is likewise difficult to treat, dehydration must be prevented. You may find this difficult if your loved one has never developed a habit of drinking water or if she is quite frail and less mobile, but there are tools and skills you can use so that you can alert her doctor that diagnosis and treatment is necessary.

There are three kinds of dehydration. Each has different causes, each requires a different type of treatment, and each poses a serious threat to your loved one.

Chart A: Three Kinds of Dehydration

TYPE	PROCESS	CAUSE	OSMOLALLITY
Isotonic	Balanced loss of water and sodium	Vomiting, diarrhea	Normal (285-295 mOsm/kg)
Hypertonic	Water losses exceed sodium losses	Fever	Increased (>300 mOsm/kg)
Hypotonic	Sodium losses exceed water losses	Overuse of diuretics	Decreased (<250mOsm/kg)

Nursing homes are required by federal law to meet residents' nutrition and hydration needs. If your loved one lives in a nursing home—even temporarily during rehabilitation following surgery or hospitalization—you will want to review these requirements in the endnotes and make sure that the staff caring for your loved one is complying with them.[1] Make no assumptions, because as my family learned, just because it's required does not mean that it's happening.

Nursing homes are required to maintain good nutrition and hydration if one of three situations prevails: (1) an existing disease process (such as terminal cancer) progresses and interferes with adequate nutrition and hydration, (2) the resident develops a new disease process in addition to the original diagnosis and it causes malnutrition and dehydration, or (3) the resident refuses food and water. If an existing disease or a new diagnosis places a resident at risk for malnutrition and dehydration, nursing homes must provide appropriate nutrition and hydration services [2] so that the resident may "attain and maintain the highest practicable physical, mental, and psychosocial well-being." This means nursing home staff must assist a resident who can no longer lift a fork, spoon, or glass to her mouth, and if a resident refuses food because she is depressed, the facility is required by law to assess the condition and provide appropriate treatment and services.

Despite federal oversight, dehydration is common in the frail elderly who live in long-term care settings. It is also common among the elderly who live in the community. In fact, the elderly aged 85 to 99 are six times[3] as likely to suffer dehydration as those aged 65 to 69.[4] Those most at risk have multiple chronic illnesses, take many dosages and/or kinds of medications, and/or have a debilitated functional status, making fluid intake difficult.[5]

Serious Consequences of Dehydration

Dehydration places the elderly at high risk of serious consequences, including the onset or worsening of delirium, disorientation, confusion, bedsores (decubitus ulcers), urinary tract infections, pneumonia, and constipation. Respiratory illness, metabolic imbalances, kidney stone formation, mitral valve prolapse, some kinds of cancer, and gastroenteritis are other conditions that can either be brought on by or exacerbated by dehydration.[6] Dehydration may also interfere with diabetes control.

More seriously, dehydration impairs kidney function and puts the patient at risk for serious consequences such as kidney failure and drug toxicity. Most drugs are excreted through the kidneys. When the kidneys fail to work properly, those drugs will remain in the bloodstream and may reach toxic levels. This is a critical problem in a frail elder who is being given many different medications. To avoid toxicity, two things should occur. First, a dehydrated patient's medications should be reduced. Second, the dehydration must be treated appropriately. Neither of these occurred with Mom. In fact, I learned that a cause of her death was "toxic encephalopathy"—brain death due to toxins. In layperson's language, Mom was poisoned by her own medicines.

Ultimately, untreated dehydration can lead to electrolyte imbalance, shock, convulsions, coma, and death. Fully 50% of those hospitalized with dehydration as the primary diagnosis will die within one year. Of those, more than 18% will die within a month of admission.[7]

To assist your loved one's caregivers in avoidance and early detection of dehydration, you will need to know the risk factors that make your loved one susceptible to it. Then you need to be aware of how to detect dehydration, how it is treated and, most importantly, how you can intervene to prevent dehydration from affecting your loved one.

There are four keys to avoiding dehydration:

- Recognizing the at-risk patient
- Observing the at-risk patient closely to detect any possible causes of dehydration
- Working with your loved one's physician to treat the factors that put her at risk for dehydration.
- Preventing dehydration in the first place

Recognizing the At-Risk Elderly Patient

To detect dehydration early, you must be aware of whether your loved one is at risk and what factors make her vulnerable to dehydration. If your loved one has any of the risk factors described below, this will compound the problem of prevention. Recognition of these risk factors is key to critical early diagnosis and treatment of dehydration. Recognition is also an important key to prevention. The factors that make your loved one at risk for dehydration include:

ADVANCED AGE

Ideally, as fluids are taken in through the mouth and excreted in various ways, including sweating, respiration, and in the urine and feces, the human body maintains a proper balance of fluids. But knowing certain facts that apply to all elderly persons can help you prevent dehydration in your elderly loved one. As people age, their kidneys have a decreased ability to concentrate urine and the body does not conserve water as well. Since older people are less likely to experience thirst, this presents a potentially serious problem since increased thirst is normally the major defense against dehydration. By the time your loved one realizes she is thirsty, she is already dehydrated.

If your loved one is like many elderly persons, she doesn't have a lifelong habit of drinking fluids and her intake has typically been substandard. As is common in the elderly, she finds maintaining a balance difficult because of age-related changes in how she metabolizes water.[8]

Advanced Age is a Risk Factor for the Elderly

Dehydration is common in the frail elderly whether they live in long-term care settings or in their own homes or the home of a family caregiver. The elderly aged 85 to 99 are six times as likely to become dehydrated as those aged 65 to 69.

INCREASED FLUID LOSSES DUE TO ILLNESS

Many illnesses result in fluid losses and lead to dehydration, including the following:

- A urinary tract infection in the previous 30 days
- Fever
- Diarrhea
- Sweating
- Internal bleeding
- Previous episodes of dehydration
- Vomiting

It is essential that fluids lost because of these conditions be replaced.

MEDICATION SIDE EFFECTS

Many medications can put the elderly at risk for dehydration because their side effects, such as drowsiness or loss of appetite, cause a decrease in fluid intake. If your loved one takes numerous medications, she may be more at risk for dehydration.

A side effect of some medications is anorexia (loss of appetite). Antipsychotics may cause your loved one to become dehydrated because they cause sedation. If your loved one's medications cause her to be sleepy, she may simply forget to drink fluids. Also, some of her fluid intake occurs as she eats since many foods contain significant fluid. If your loved one decreases her food intake, her fluid intake will also be reduced.

You will want to check to see whether any of your loved one's medications can cause dysphagia—difficulty in swallowing. Researchers find that many elderly persons suffer from undiagnosed dysphagia. Other medications cause delirium, the mental confusion you learned about in Chapter Two, and dystonia, a side effect discussed in Chapter Four. All of these conditions will make it difficult for your loved one to drink. You'll find many helpful tools in the appendices to help you keep track of her medications and their side effects.

DECREASED FLUID INTAKE

The recommended amount of fluids is between 30 to 35 mL/kg per day, or six to eight eight-ounce glasses.[9] If your loved one is fearful of urinary incontinence, she may purposefully restrict fluids to avoid having "an accident" when she has to rush to the toilet. Unless she consumes at least 75% of the recommended amount of fluids, she is at risk for dehydration. In a 1999 study, Burger found that only one in 40 nursing home residents observed drank sufficient fluids.[10]

CONFUSION AND LOSS OF MOBILITY

If your loved one is confused or suffers from dementia or delirium, she is at risk for dehydration, because she will often fail to recognize thirst and/or adequately care for her hydration needs. If she suffers a loss of mobility or has problems with dizziness or vertigo, she is as much at risk for dehydration as one who has comprehension or communication problems. She may fail to drink adequate fluids because she afraid of falling and thus does not get up independently to get herself a drink of water.

INABILITY TO FEED ONESELF

Many foods contain significant amounts of fluid. Your loved one takes in water in foods such as soups, broths, fruits, and Jell-O. If she finds it impossible to feed herself and if she is dependent upon aides at meals, she is at far greater risk for dehydration. As Burger and her colleagues discovered, understaffing in nursing homes leads to inadequate and/or ineffective feeding for many of these functionally impaired persons. (Understaffing is covered in detail in Chapter Eight.) If your loved one has hand dexterity problems or body control problems, is bed-bound, has swallowing problems or dysphagia, or requires intravenous fluids, she is at risk for dehydration as a result of an impaired ability to feed herself.

Your loved one is also very vulnerable to dehydration if she must be fed by an aide. Keeping in mind that it takes 30 to 60 minutes to feed a person safely and efficiently, it becomes quite clear that there are often too few staff members available in nursing homes to enable all the residents to receive the assistance in eating they require.[11]

ADDITIONAL RISK FACTORS

Additional risk factors for dehydration include illnesses that are accompanied by vomiting, fever, or diarrhea because fluids are lost from the body as a result. Other risk factors include eating poorly (25% of food left uneaten at most meals), failure to take medication(s), or rapid weight loss. According to Burger, physicians writing for the American Medical Association consider a rapid weight loss of greater than three% in a 28-day period to be a trigger for evaluation of dehydration.[12]

Detecting Dehydration

Early detection of dehydration depends on careful monitoring of nutritional intake, both food and fluids, which should be reviewed on a daily basis. If your loved one consistently takes in fluids of 1500 cc (about six to eight cups) or less each day, you should be especially alert to the potential for dehydration. Dehydration in an older person is not easily recognized, particularly in the early stages, but there are ways you can help detect it in your loved one so that you can seek prompt intervention.

OBSERVABLE SIGNS

Dizziness and irregular heartbeat as well as constipation, lethargy, delirium, and confusion can be caused by dehydration and thus may be indicators of dehydration. Other early signs and symptoms of dehydration include headache, fatigue, and heat intolerance. Dryness in the mouth or eyes is another sign.

While urine color darkens as dehydration develops because it becomes concentrated, this is not a sensitive indicator for early dehydration. By the time your loved one has concentrated urine, she is probably already in the later stages of dehydration.

Weight loss is another indicator of dehydration. One pound of body weight is equal to 455 mL of water; a weight loss of three pounds is an indicator of dehydration. (Three pounds is equal to 1365 mL. This is about eight cups or one-half gallon and is the amount of fluids an adult should drink each day.)

Observable Signs and Symptoms of Dehydration

Dizziness
Irregular heartbeat
Constipation
Lethargy
Delirium
Confusion
Weight loss (> 3% in 28 days)
Headache
Fatigue
Heat intolerance
Dryness in the mouth or eyes

LABORATORY TESTS

Laboratory test results can help make a diagnosis of dehydration. Keep in mind that because abnormal values are "normal" for some people, it is important to look for changes in values.

Electrolyte imbalance. Monitoring electrolyte imbalance is critical in detecting dehydration in your loved one.[13] Do not, as I did, underestimate the serious threat this poses for her. If electrolytes are not perfectly balanced in the body, many organs, including the heart, cannot function properly. If you've ever watched college football on TV, you'll remember that athletes consume large quantities of Gatorade. This is a fluid that is specially formulated to prevent electrolyte imbalances from occurring as the players lose copious fluids through perspiration during their play, particularly on hot days. In fact, on very hot days, when electrolyte imbalances may occur, you may remember seeing players suffering muscle cramps or spasms so intense they limped from the field, not to return until after fluid replacements. I've even seen games on very hot days where the TV commentators reported that some players were taken to the locker room and given intravenous fluids! Electrolyte imbalances are a very serious problem indeed. Keep in mind that if your loved one develops an electrolyte imbalance and it remains untreated, her condition will be fatal.

I knew nothing about electrolyte imbalance before Mom died. I've since learned that her electrolyte imbalance, diagnosed but never treated, was the precipitating factor in all of the complications that led to her death. The following explanation is intended to help you avoid a similar occurrence in your loved one. [Details more harrowing and complicated are found in endnote 15 for this chapter.]

Alpine Manor had written on Mom's few records sent to the Traverse City facility that she had an electrolyte disorder. This didn't mean anything to me, and Alpine Manor's staff did not seem concerned about it. They never mentioned it when I asked them about the drastic changes in Mom's condition, nor did they mention it when I picked Mom up to take her to Traverse City. One piece of paper had hand-written lab test results, but no one noticed that these results were from October 13 instead of November 6. We all knew that Alpine Manor had done tests on November 6 just before the transfer, and we assumed those were the test results we were given. Mom's internist in mid-Michigan noted the electrolyte imbalance but did not seem overly concerned, so I had no idea this was a life-threatening condition.

After Mom's death, I found a diagnosis of acute electrolyte imbalance in her discharge record and autopsy report.[14] As I researched electrolyte imbalance, the term "osmolality" appeared. Osmolality is the concentration of particles of electrolytes in solution and is determined by examining the fluid portion of a blood sample in the lab. Osmolality increases with dehydration (the number of particles increases) and decreases with overhydration. It is determined by measuring the ratio of sodium, potassium, urea, and glucose.

Physicians use a complicated mathematical formula to make this determination, but you don't need to be a doctor or nurse to monitor your loved one's status. To help you detect dehydration in its early stages so that you can alert physicians and nurses that treatment is needed, you simply need to keep track of the lab tests your loved one has, tests her physician will call "an electrolyte panel." Keep a chart with the lab values for sodium (Na), Potassium (K), urea (BUN), and glucose. You can plug these values into a calculator on an Internet website to determine her osmolality. This calculator is found at www.intmed.mcw.edu/clincalc/osmol.html. If the calculation you make exceeds the normal range (normal osmolality is 285 to 295),[15] you should contact her physician's office immediately.

Although there are other simpler ways to detect dehydration, which will be discussed below, calculating osmolality provides a more accurate assessment for those who are able to use this method of detecting dehydration.

Kidney function. Monitoring kidney function is critical to the detection and management of dehydration and can be done in several ways. Perhaps the easiest way is to look at BUN and serum creatinine levels. According to Dr. John E. Morley, a ratio greater than 20:1 is highly suggestive of dehydration.[16] If regular lab tests are available for your loved one, BUN and serum creatinine levels will be readily available to you. Divide the value for BUN that you find on your loved one's lab tests by the value you find for serum creatinine (SCr). If the number you get is greater than 20, call her doctor right away.

Another way you can monitor kidney function is to calculate creatinine clearance.[17] While it is possible for physicians to get a lab test to determine creatinine clearance, the test usually takes 24 hours. It is important to detect kidney failure quickly, so physicians often use a formula to estimate creatinine clearance. In other words, they measure how effectively the kidneys are filtering out creatinine, which tells them how well the kidneys are functioning. Although this is a somewhat complicated matter, you don't need to know how or why it works. All you need to do is plug a few numbers—values from your loved one's most recent lab tests—into a different online calculator. If the calculator indicates there is a problem, you will need to alert your loved one's physicians and nurses immediately because early detection and treatment is key to survival.

You will need to know your loved one's weight, age, and serum creatinine (SCr on her lab tests). Plug these numbers into the calculator at www.intmed.mcw.edu/clincalc/creatinine.html. If the number you get—the estimated creatinine clearance—is lower than 50 to 55, you should alert her medical team members right away.

What Does Low Creatinine Clearance Mean?

Impaired creatinine clearance is indicative of the following:

- Kidney damage due to drug toxicity
- Damage to the structure of the kidney, which will lead to kidney failure
- Dehydration
- Congestive heart failure
- Obstruction of urine in the kidney
- Shock
- Acute or chronic kidney failure
- End-stage renal disease

Because a failure to treat these conditions will lead to death, it is important that kidney function be monitored, that drug dosages be decreased or eliminated in the event of an impairment in kidney function, and that aggressive treatment of the underlying condition be promptly initiated.

According to Joel Shuster, professor of clinical pharmacy at Temple University School of Pharmacy, normal kidney function for most elderly persons is a glomerular filtration rate (GFR) of 50-55 to 70-75 mL/min.[18] (85-125 mL/min is normal for a young adult.) When kidneys are functioning below a GFR level of 10, a person needs dialysis to remove toxins from the blood and to permit life to continue. According to Shuster, when your loved one's GFR is below 50, her medications must be thoroughly evaluated and reduced to avoid the risk for toxicity that can be fatal. If you find information that your loved one's kidney function is faltering, it is very appropriate and necessary for you to ask her physician whether she might reduce or eliminate some medications, particularly those with side effects that might have had a negative impact on your loved one's kidney function.

Use the tools in Appendix L to keep track of your loved one's BUN to creatinine ratio and also her GFR.

Weight loss. As mentioned above, you should consider a weight loss of three% as a trigger for considering the possibility of dehydration. Weight loss may be one of the easiest things to monitor if you are able to make sure your loved one is weighed consistently on a weekly basis (or more frequently if her status is very fragile). Be aware that experts consider this the least reliable method.

One other method sometimes used involves lifting a pinch of skin on the patient's arm using your thumb and forefinger to examine elasicity. I remember clearly that when Mom and I were in Dr. Scott's office just before we left for Traverse City, I expressed concern that Mom was dehydrated. Dr. Scott's nurse did this skin test and assured me that Mom was not dehydrated. It was long after Mom's death that I learned about osmolality and realized how critically dehydrated she was on that day. I can tell you from personal experience not to trust this very unscientific and subjective method of detecting dehydration.

Treating Dehydration

If your loved one develops dehydration, you will need to understand the various kinds of treatment. As shown in Chart A at the beginning of this chapter, there are three kinds of dehydration, so treatment will depend upon which type of dehydration your loved one has.

ISOTONIC DEHYDRATION

Isotonic dehydration is due to a balanced loss of water and sodium, typically resulting from total abstinence of food and water or a large volume loss from diarrhea or vomiting. Electrolyte concentrations remain near normal. Loss of volume without electrolyte disturbance constitutes the simplest type of dehydration. In this case, treatment consists of replacing the volume deficit over 24 hours.

HYPERTONIC DEHYDRATION

In hypertonia, loss of water is greater than loss of sodium. Fever can precipitate hypertonia, although excess sweating may also cause this condition. Signs of hypertonia include warm, doughy, velvety skin, dry mucous membranes, muscular signs such as twitching and hyperreflexia (an exaggeration of reflexes), and central nervous system symptoms such as lethargy, confusion, irritability, rigidity, generalized convulsions, and finally, coma. To treat hypertonia, the serum sodium concentration must be corrected slowly over at least 48 hours.

The goal is to avoid dropping the sodium too quickly. It is not unusual for total body sodium to be below normal, and this must be corrected as well.

HYPOTONIC DEHYDRATION

Hypotonic dehydration is defined as sodium loss exceeding water loss. This type of fluid disturbance is most often due to use of diuretics. Hypotonic dehydration primarily affects the central nervous system (CNS) and musculoskeletal systems. CNS effects include headache, fatigue, anorexia, lethargy, confusion, disorientation, agitation, vomiting, seizures, and coma. Musculoskeletal symptoms may include cramps and weakness. Hypontonia is fairly severe if these symptoms are present.

If your loved one is hypotonic, diuretics should be discontinued and fluid replacement should be carefully initiated. Hypertonicity must be corrected slowly, for she may be harmed if fluids are introduced too quickly. If, however, she is displaying signs of central nervous system (CNS) involvement or is experiencing seizures, a partial correction of the sodium deficit can be achieved rapidly. The danger of drug toxicity is serious.

Your loved one should receive intravenous fluids as soon as possible after a diagnosis of dehydration. One method that can be used at home or in nursing homes is subcutaneous infusion, which means injecting fluids under the skin in a place with lots of skin area, usually the stomach or thighs.[19] Since this method does not require an IV, which may not be available in nursing homes that do not offer skilled care, its use may eliminate the need for hospitalization.

Since a large amount of fluids are provided by food, if your loved one is dehydrated, you may have to address whether tube feeding is required. This is a difficult question and one that many families wish to avoid, for once tube feeding is begun it is difficult if not impossible to make a decision to discontinue it. Tube feeding is discussed more fully in Chapters Seven and Nine.

Obviously, it is best to avoid dehydration altogether. This is most feasible if you or another family caregiver takes responsibility for consistently monitoring your loved one's condition.

Preventing Dehydration

To prevent dehydration, do the following:

ASSESSMENT

- Ask your loved one's physician to evaluate her medications, the specific medications and also the dosages, and to consider reduction, substitution, or elimination of medications in light of her kidney function as determined by electrolyte or other testing or observable side effects that restrict her ability to take in fluids.

- Ask her physician to assess her in light of confusion or dementia to determine how capable your loved one is of providing herself with adequate liquids and of appreciating thirst and the need for fluid intake.

- You may need to have an occupational or physical therapist make an assessment of physical problems that can impact your loved one's ability to drink fluids. For example, if she has difficulty swallowing, a speech therapist should evaluate her swallowing function.

OBSERVATION

- Observe your loved one at mealtimes and when drinking if her intake is consistently poor to identify the problem and also to document intake.

- Learn your loved one's fluid preferences, communicate them to the staff, and offer fluids she prefers.

ASSISTANCE

- Make sure your loved one has access to fluids and do not rely on thirst to prompt fluid intake, because most elderly individuals perceive thirst poorly, if at all.

- Be aware of your loved one's physical limitations. You may need to offer physical assistance in drinking fluids or you may need to provide adaptive glasses or cups.

- Offer electrolyte-replacing solutions such as Gatorade instead of water if hyponatremia (dehydration with an electrolyte imbalance) is a problem. Try freezing one of these solutions into Popsicles for your loved one.

- Be attentive to the fluid requirements if your loved one is confused or delirious, for she will lack the ability to understand that she needs to drink fluids.

- If your loved one is at risk for aspiration pneumonia, fluids may need to be introduced in other ways. For example, applesauce, puddings, and Jell-O may be used for fluid intake if swallowing thin liquids is too difficult.

- Thickett, a product that can be ordered without a prescription through a drug store, will enable you to thicken liquids and runny foods to a consistency that is easier for her to swallow.
- Find out what staff members will be alerted and available to help her. Follow up to make sure she is getting that help.

ENCOURAGEMENT

- Encourage fluid intake by offering ice chips, Popsicles, juice bars, gelatin, ice cream, sherbet, soup, broth, fruits, fruit and vegetable juices, lemonade, and flavored water.

SPECIAL CAUTIONS

- Offer supplemental fluids to your loved one if she is vomiting, has diarrhea, a fever, or is receiving diuretics, as she will be losing more fluids than normal.
- Remember that each degree of fever adds an additional 300 cc's daily to your loved one's fluid requirement.
- Avoid coffee and alcohol, which are diuretics.
- Do not use straws if your loved one has chewing and swallowing problems. Straws increase air swallowing and add to the number of steps required for drinking.

Because of dehydration's potentially fatal consequences, you will want to take an active role in helping your loved one's medical team watch for signs of it, do the assessments to detect it, and, most of all, to prevent it.

CHAPTER SEVEN

Malnutrition: A Serious Problem for the Institutionalized Elderly As Well As Those at Home

NOVEMBER 6, 2000

Glen and I arrived at Alpine Manor at about noon to pick Mom up and transfer her to the extended care facility in Traverse City. I found her in the day room, sitting at a table for people who needed assistance in eating from an aide.

An aide was feeding the woman next to Mom. Someone had thrown a bib on the table in front of Mom but had not put it on her. Mom had a plate of food in front of her and was trying to feed herself. Her plate held a piece of fish and some potatoes. A bowl of large whole Brussels sprouts was on her right. Mom was stabbing repeatedly at the fish, trying to get a piece of food onto her fork. It was obvious that she had been attempting to eat for a while because the front of her shirt was soiled with food.

I was horrified at the sight of my mom, who was trying helplessly and unsuccessfully to feed herself, while the aide simply watched her and made no effort to help. I met the eyes of the aide. Her eyes carried this message: "Yeah, so what are you going to do about it?"

I asked Mom if I could help her eat. She indicated that she just wanted to go. I collected her discharge papers from the social worker, who had already told me a staff doctor was going to be signing Mom out because her attending physician had not seen her at all in the seven weeks she had been there.

The social worker also told me they had done lab work on Mom that day but they had been unable to do a urine test. Despite the lack of a urine culture, they were prescribing an antibiotic for seven days because they thought she had a urinary tract infection. Other prescriptions for Mom's usual medications were also ready. The antipsychotic was not on her list of medications, but I knew she'd been given it as recently as November 4, according to the pre-registration records that had been telefaxed to the new facility.

I proceeded to check Mom out. The discharge sheet said that she was able to walk with a walker, to propel her own wheelchair, and to eat 75% of the food on her plate. It also said that she weighed 115 pounds. None of this was true.

I asked for a cup of chipped ice so that I could keep Mom's mouth moistened and it was prepared for me. The social worker assisted Glen and me in transferring Mom from the wheelchair to our vehicle.

Before we drove Mom to Traverse City, I took her to the office of Dr. Scott, her personal physician who had cared for her for years. I had made her an appointment in the belief that her own internist would be in a better position to assist the Traverse City medical personnel in evaluating what was wrong.

I asked the nurse who did the intake about dehydration. After a brief physical examination that included testing the skin tone, she said she did not think Mom was dehydrated.

Dr. Scott, Mom's physician, was a warm, pleasant, and energetic Scottish lady. She was puzzled and concerned about the great change in Mom's condition since she'd seen her two months earlier. She mentioned the electrolyte imbalance, though she did not seem alarmed by it. She told me that she would be willing to assist Mom's new physician in Traverse City and told me to have him telephone her if he wanted more information.

Mom had been quiet during this exam. Suddenly she looked up and said, "Have a good vacation." The doctor, apparently thinking Mom had asked if she'd had a good vacation, smiled and told Mom about her recent trip with Doctors Without Borders. Then she left the room and Mom looked at me and asked, "When are you leaving?"

Mom knew we were scheduled to leave for Florida in November. Remembering a conversation in August when she had tearfully told me that she did not want to be a burden to anyone, I realized that she was concerned her illness would interfere with our vacation. I assured her that everything would be okay—that I would not go away soon and that I would not go if she needed me. I did not know these were the last words I would hear from Mom.

We drove to Traverse City and got Mom settled in for the night. About 10:30 p.m., the telephone rang. It was Jill, telling me that Dr. Scott wanted to talk with me and that it was okay to telephone her now, that she was expecting a call from me.

When I reached her, Dr. Scott told me that she'd been thinking about her examination of Mom and that she wanted me to tell Dr. John, my physician and now Mom's, to schedule Mom for a complete neurological workup—that there was something wrong. I wrote a memo to telefax to Dr. John's office in the morning. In retrospect, of course, I should have taken Mom to his office rather than to the nursing home and requested that he admit her to the hospital.

He eventually ordered the work-up, but by that time, it was all very much too late.

A registered nurse stayed with Mom that evening, feeding her, giving her liquids, and watching over her in the night. Mom ate little, the nurse reported in the morning, and she had been fairly delirious. How I wish I'd known enough then to take Mom to the hospital instead of to the nursing home.

Malnutrition—An Epidemic

Malnourishment, also referred to here as protein-energy malnutrition or PEM, is epidemic among the elderly, regardless of where they live. In 1998, Dr. John E. Morley, a noted geriatrics practitioner and long-term care nutritionist, cautioned that 40% of U.S. nursing facility residents are malnourished, 44% of home health patients are malnourished, and 50% of hospital patients are malnourished. [1]

It would be a mistake to assume that malnutrition is caused by poverty. While poverty is sometimes a factor, many common conditions affecting the elderly contribute to malnutrition. These include the normal effects of aging on the body, including an impaired appetite and a decline in the ability to smell and taste food; medical, environmental, economic, and social problems; and poor oral health, whether decay, gum disease, ill-fitting dentures, or other problems. Many things that cause malnutrition are the same things that cause ADRs, falls, and dehydration. Age-related changes in absorption of food and in ability to eat quantities of food also affect nutrition.

PEM Is Epidemic Among the Elderly

The rate of PEM in nursing homes compares with that of poverty-stricken third-world countries.[2]

In June of 2000, Burger and her colleagues published a major indictment of nursing home care, "Malnutrition and Dehydration in Nursing Homes: Key Issues in Prevention and Treatment," under the auspices of the National Citizen's Coalition for Nursing Home Reform.[3] Her report cited studies saying that 35% of nursing home residents suffer from malnutrition or under-nutrition and she cited other studies with much higher rates—up to 85%![4]

The consequences of PEM are dire. PEM creates significant risk that existing diseases and conditions will worsen, that new ones will develop, and that death will occur. People suffering from malnutrition have a higher incidence of concurrent illnesses such as pneumonia. If your malnourished loved one is hospitalized, she'll be about five times as likely to die when compared with well-nourished patients. There are many reasons for this. When people are malnourished, they get more infections and diseases, their injuries take longer to heal, and surgery on them is riskier.[5]

Malnutrition is preventable, but it often goes undiagnosed. Like dehydration, it is difficult to reverse and may be fatal. Therefore, prevention is critical. You can help to ensure that your loved one gets proper nutrition, whether she lives in the community or in a nursing facility, but it is more difficult to provide this service than it may first appear.

UNDERSTANDING MALNUTRITION AND HOW THE BODY WORKS

How nutrition works is a pretty complicated subject, but it boils down to this: your loved one needs Calories (i.e., carbohydrates and fat) to make energy and she needs protein in order to synthesize tissue. Ideally, Calories are "burned off" or expended by exercise. Otherwise, the excess Calories are stored as fat.

According to Dr. Demling, the idea that the frail elderly slow down metabolically and require less nutrition is a myth. In fact, the elderly require at least 25% more calories than the standard recommended daily allowance (RDA) tables recommend for adults just to avoid losing lean mass, bone, calcium, and to avoid chronic conditions such as diminished cognition and adult onset diabetes. This is problematic, because the elderly typically do not eat properly. According to Demling, the elderly require 1 to 1.2 grams of protein per kilogram per day *just to maintain* lean body mass, and also require supplemental calcium and vitamin D to avoid or decrease osteoporosis. They need vitamin B complex and folic acid to counteract increases in homocysteine and to protect heart function.[6] All this is just to *maintain* function, not to restore lost function or tissue.

It might be helpful to think of the healing process as a kind of "battle" that pits the body's normal digestive process against the wound healing. The body wants protein to maintain its status. The wound wants protein to rebuild tissue. Surgery, bedsores, a broken hip, and illness or infection that has destroyed body tissue all can be considered "wounds."

In response to illness, injury, or infection, the body's hormones activate a "flight or fright" stress reaction. Inflammation occurs, either at the site of a wound or generally in the body. This stimulates an unhealthy kind of metabolism called "catabolism" and tissue breaks down as protein breaks down.[7]

As a result, the body's demand for energy increases dramatically and the way that nutrients are used changes. The body begins to use protein for energy, instead of using it to build tissue. The body actually begins feeding upon itself, using protein or lean body mass for fuel. One author calls this "auto-cannibalism."[8]

When, in response to a stressed condition, the body breaks down its own lean body mass in order to survive, muscle mass is lost and the immune system and organ function are impaired. Severely malnourished persons become weak, fatigued, and apathetic. They tend to stay in bed and refuse to eat. If not treated, they die.

The rate at which protein is consumed is astonishing. If your loved one suffers a broken hip, for example, the catabolism activated by her hormonal response to her injury could result in a loss of one to two pounds of lean body mass per day, depending both upon the strength of her catabolism and how much nutritional support she is given. Indeed, when catabolism, PEM, aging, or illness are present, up to 30% of consumed protein is used for energy. This destructive trend in her metabolism would only be reversed after her injury has healed and the metabolic rate returns to normal. If your loved one's metabolic process was compromised before her injury, and if as a result your loved one develops PEM during the healing process, reversal will be very slow.[9]

What Factors Make Your Loved One at Risk for Malnutrition?

If your loved one lives in a nursing home, you should be aware that she is at particular risk for PEM. She will be most at risk if she is acutely injured, chronically ill, incapacitated, unable to think logically, or is functionally impaired. If your loved one is unable to feed herself or to recognize hunger, she will also be at increased risk for death by malnutrition.

Morley and his associates developed the mnemonic MEALS-ON-WHEELS to designate the most common, treatable causes of malnutrition.[10] You can use the following list to help your loved one's physicians and nurses determine early on whether your loved one is at risk for malnutrition. According to Morley, the first two causes of PEM, medications and depression, are the most prevalent.

- Medications
- Emotional problems (depression)
- Anorexia (from disease processes, drugs, or emotional problems), alcoholism
- Late-life paranoia (rare)
- Swallowing disorders (e.g., dysphagia)
- Oral factors (e.g., poor dental health, gum infections, ill-fitting dentures)
- Nosocomial infections (hospital-caused infections)
- Wandering and other dementia-related behaviors (i.e., the resident fails to recognize hunger or the need to eat)
- Hyperthyroidism, hypercalcemia, hypoadrenalism
- Enteral problems (malabsorption)
- Eating problems (e.g., the inability to feed oneself)
- Low-salt, low cholesterol diets (resulting in foods that aren't taste-tempting)
- Stones (gallstones)

MEDICATIONS MAY INCREASE YOUR LOVED ONE'S RISK FOR MALNUTRITION

Many drugs have harmful side effects such as anorexia, nausea and vomiting, diarrhea, the inability to think logically, or increased metabolism[11] that can lead to malnutrition. If your loved one takes an average of three or more drugs per day, she's at high risk for malnutrition.[12]

To protect your loved one, you'll need to know which drugs are most likely to adversely affect her and to result in nutritional decline. They are:

- Digoxin (used to treat heart problems such as heart failure and atrial fibrillation)
- Antipsychotics (used to treat some mental illnesses such as schizophrenia and psychosis)
- Benzodiazepines (used to treat anxiety)
- Antidepressants
- Hypnotics
- Diuretics (used to treat water retention problems)
- NSAIDs (non-steroidal anti-inflammatory medications such as aspirin, Motrin, Advil)
- Anticonvulsants

These medications affect your loved one's nutritional status in various ways. Specifically, Digoxin, used to treat heart arrhythmias, can cause anorexia, nausea, and vomiting. These conditions may result in a reduction in protein-calorie intake.

Antipsychotics and other psychoactive medications may cause her to have a disinterest in food and drink.[13]

Be particularly wary of diuretics, which can cause alterations in kidney function. As a result, minerals and salts essential to body function—sodium, potassium, zinc, and magnesium—may be lost.

Aspirin may cause silent gastrointestinal blood loss, inducing iron deficiency and anemia.

NSAIDs inhibit the absorption of calcium and also alter how glucose is metabolized. Various harmful conditions can result including osteoporosis, hyperglycemia, increased levels of sodium, and decreased levels of potassium.

Anti-seizure medications such as phenobarbital act upon the central nervous system and alter enzymes in the liver, resulting in changes in vitamin D metabolism.

Even over-the-counter medications can cause drug-nutrient interactions. For example, use of a mineral oil laxative can inhibit fat-soluble vitamin absorption and lead to malabsorption of vitamins A, D, E, and K.[14]

Additionally, medications can alter metabolism, increasing losses of nutrients and creating vitamin or mineral deficiencies.

The following medications can also increase your loved one's risk for malnutrition. Talk to your loved one's doctor if she takes any of these:

- Antacids
- H_2 blockers (medications used to prevent the production of stomach acid)
- Anti-neoplastic agents (tumor-suppressing drugs)
- Hypoglycemic agents (used to maintain blood sugar levels)

CHRONIC CONDITIONS AND DISEASES CAUSE PEM

You'll also need to be watchful for malnutrition if your loved one suffers chronic conditions and illnesses. Some conditions negatively affect taste or smell, making food less palatable. Delirium or dementia can impair your loved one's awareness of hunger. Your loved one may eat improperly because she finds it difficult or impossible to fix or eat a balanced diet or because she develops food idiosyncrasies and limits her diet to one or more specific foods. Lack of information or knowledge may lead your loved one to make poor choices in food. She might, for example, get in a rut—refuse to eat anything other than certain "comfort foods." If she suddenly decides that she wants nothing other than tomato soup with oyster crackers, then her meals contain no protein. You'll want to supervise her nutritional intake to make sure it is adequate in terms of quality as well as quantity, and that she eats well-balanced meals.[15]

You'll also want to assess your loved one's risk for malnutrition in light of the following conditions common in the elderly, all of which contribute to the development of anorexia and malnutrition: dementia, pain, immobility, reflux, constipation, alcoholism, drug addiction, polypharmacy (use of three or more prescribed drugs), dental problems, xerostomia (dry mouth), alterations in hunger or thirst recognition, and impaired taste.

Unrecognized and untreated dysphagia (difficulty in swallowing) may lead to malnutrition, dehydration, asphyxiation, and aspiration pneumonia.[16] Because dysphagia has such dire consequences and is so prevalent, with nearly 50% of the elderly suffering from it to some degree, you'll want to be sure it is evaluated as a cause of malnutrition for your loved one and treated if it's diagnosed. You will find a checklist to help you detect dysphagia and its causes in Appendix M.

The following conditions and diseases are also often implicated in the development of malnutrition:[17]

Neurological (central nervous system) disorders:
- Parkinson's disease
- Head trauma

Psychological disorders:
- Depression (a most common precipitator of PEM)

Metabolic disorders:
- Diabetes mellitus
- Addison's disease
- Hypothyroidism

Systemic disorders:
- Cirrhosis of the liver
- Cancer
- Chronic renal failure
- Zinc deficiency

- Intestinal tract diseases impairing absorption
- Cardiovascular disease
- Chronic obstructive pulmonary disease

Catabolic illness:
- Trauma
- Surgery
- Wounds
- Infection
- Corticosteroids

Environmental conditions:
- Rhinitis
- Sinusitis
- Radiation

Detecting Protein/Energy Malnutrition

PEM, which is usually slow in developing, initially presents as fatigue. Your loved one may then experience progressive weight loss that is in fact a loss of both fat and lean mass.

According to the Nutrition Screening Initiative, a group collaborative effort of family physicians, the American Dietetic Association and the National Council on Aging, if you see any of the following in your loved one, you will want to alert her medical caregivers to your concerns about whether they would support a diagnosis of malnutrition:[19]

Body weight

- Has lost five pounds or 5% of weight in one month
- Has lost 10 pounds or 10% of weight in the past six months
- Body mass index is <24[20]

Assessment should be based on your loved one's "normal" weight, not her weight just prior to being a wound patient, because weight loss has likely already occurred.[21]

Keep track of your loved one's weight so that you're aware of her status and any changes in it. Keep in mind that appearances are not usually a good indicator of weight loss, since you may not see your loved one except when she is dressed and weight loss is not readily discernible. Consequently, be sure your loved one is regularly weighed, at approximately the same time of day, and that she wears similar clothing while being weighed to ensure greater accuracy. Keep notes in your records of your loved one's weight, being sure you have weekly records.

More important, rely on your loved one's BMI, or Body Mass Index, as the true measuring stick for detecting malnutrition. BMI is the most sensitive measurement of nutritional status. When BMI is used, 31% of elderly patients are identified as malnourished, whereas only 8% are identified as undernourished if weight loss is used as the determinant.[22]

If you can monitor your loved one's BMI, you'll be assured of being able to initiate an earlier intervention if your loved one develops PEM. In addition, you'll get better results and her recovery will be more easily assured.[23] You can use the materials in Appendix L to help you monitor your loved one's nutritional status. There, you'll not only find the URLs for the calculators on the Internet that will help you monitor her status, you'll also find the URL for a calculator to help you calculate her BMI and a chart to use to keep track of increases or decreases in her BMI.

Some studies in medical journals recommend much more conservative triggers for dangerously low BMIs than the numbers presented above.[24] Since using more conservative numbers will lead to earlier detection and intervention, you may want to follow their lead. These studies evaluate women differently from men instead of "one size fits all," and have shown that there is a marked increased in mortality risk with these numbers:

For men, a BMI less than 23.5 kg/m^2

For women, a BMI less than 22 kg/m^2

Knowing these critical threshold numbers is important for you as a caregiver. If you use these more conservative numbers as your trigger for concern, rather than the federal guidelines of BMI of 19 kg/m2 that nursing homes are supposed to adhere to, your loved one's likelihood of surviving or avoiding PEM will be greatly increased. If your loved one weighs less than 100 pounds, however, the usual formula for measuring BMI simply doesn't apply. Such a low weight requires greater caution and thus you'll want to use an even higher BMI as a trigger—for example 23 kg/m^2 (for women) or 24.5 kg/m^2 (for men).

Here are the other potential red flags to be alert for.

Physical signs

- Muscle wasting
- Loss of subcutaneous fat
- Obvious loss of tissue in the face or buttocks
- Sparse, dull hair
- Orthostatic hypotension (light-headedness)
- Edema
- Poor wound healing, unhealed pressure sores, skin breakdown
- Anemia
- Cognitive impairment (difficulty with logical thinking)
- Heart failure (i.e., tachycardia, tachypnea, high or low blood pressure, edema)
- Signs of central nervous system depression or congestive heart failure
- Tongue atrophying (indicating a folate B12 deficiency)
- Cracking at the edges of the mouth (cheilitis)
- Chronic infections
- Listlessness or apathy
- Dry conjunctiva[25]

Eating habits

- Does not have enough food to eat each day
- Usually eats alone
- Does not eat anything on one or more days each month
- Has poor appetite
- Is on a special diet
- Eats vegetables two or fewer times daily
- Consumes milk or milk products once or not at all daily
- Consumes fruit or fruit juice once or not at all daily
- Eats breads, cereals, pasta, rice, or other grains five or fewer times daily
- Has difficulty chewing or swallowing
- Has more than one alcoholic drink per day if female; more than two drinks per day if male
- Has pain in mouth, teeth, or gums

Living environment

* Lives on an income of <$6,000 per year per individual
  in the household
* Lives alone
* Is housebound
* Is concerned about home security
* Lives in a home with inadequate heating or cooling
* Does not have a stove and/or refrigerator
* Is unable or prefers not to spend money on food (<$25–$30
  per person spent on food each week)

Functional status

Usually or always needs assistance with any of the following:
* Bathing
* Dressing
* Grooming
* Toileting
* Eating
* Walking or moving about
* Traveling (outside the home)
* Preparing food
* Shopping for food or other necessities

MININUTRITIONAL ASSESSMENT

One additional tool you can use to help detect and/or avoid malnutrition in your loved one is the MiniNutritional Assessment (MNA®). This screening and assessment tool was developed by Nestle and leading international geriatricians and can be accessed on the Internet. The major advantage of the MNA is that it does not use laboratory tests. Therefore, it's not only cost effective, it's something you as a family caregiver can use to evaluate your loved one's status even if you don't have access to lab tests. The Mini Nutritional Assessment may be downloaded in a .pdf file at www.mna-elderly.com/practice/user_guide/mna_guide.pdf. Last accessed March 1, 2006.

For further information and helpful guidelines, see the American Dietetic Association and the Gerontological Society of America's publication called "Clinical Guide to Prevent and Manage Malnutrition in Long-

Term Care." This helpful document can be accessed on the Internet at www.semer.org/docs/ENL-PRO-NUT.pdf Last accessed March 1, 2006.

Resolving Malnutrition

If you suspect your loved one is malnourished, you might ask her physician whether she will involve other medical caregivers in the investigation to detect and address the underlying cause or causes. Sometimes, a team consisting of physicians, nurses, dieticians, pharmacologists, physical and occupational therapists, social workers, and family members will work together to get to the bottom of your loved one's nutritional issues before malnutrition becomes a life-threatening condition.

It takes many differently trained professionals to come up with the answers, and there are several reasons for that. For one, solutions may not be medically based. If your loved one has a physical disability or suffers from Alzheimer's or anorexia, the solution may be as simple as scheduling a mealtime visit from a staff person or arranging for help in feeding.

If your loved one has dysphagia, a careful assessment will be required so that her diet may be altered to accommodate her swallowing difficulties.

If your loved one lives alone in her own home, loneliness may be a root cause of her nutritional decline as she may skip meals because eating alone isn't interesting. You might arrange for meals to be delivered by Meals on Wheels, an organization whose mission is to provide hot mid-day meals for homebound elders. Often, the person delivering meals will sit and socialize at mealtime, which may be all that is required to encourage your loved one's adequate nutrition.

If you can't identify social or environmental issues as a root cause for your loved one's nutritional decline, you should consider a new set of possible causes. Remember that one of her medications may be a potential cause, and that a change in medication may be required. At this point, you might ask your loved one's team of professionals if they will consider laboratory testing to determine if her weight loss has resulted in abnormal values. If values are abnormal, more aggressive treatment options should be pursued, since toxins may be building up in her body.

HOW YOU CAN HELP YOUR LOVED ONE HEAL AND AVOID MALNUTRITION

As a caregiver, you'll have to put a great deal of thought and effort into helping your loved one improve her diet and her food intake so that her wound-healing rate increases and she doesn't develop PEM.

Where your loved one's goal is to restore lost lean body mass to rebuild damaged tissue—heal pressure sores or a broken hip, for example—she must increase her intake of calories and make sure that her protein intake is 1.5 g/kg/day to 2 g/kg/day. Weight and lean mass gains will begin only when her caloric intake is above recommended daily allowances. According to Dr. Demling, the following are the specific protein requirements for patients with specific nutritional problems.[18]

Protein Requirements

Condition	Daily Needs
Stress response	1.5 g/kg to 2 g/kg per day
Correct protein-energy malnutrition	1.5 g/kg per day
Presence of wound	1.5 g/kg per day
Restore lost weight	1.5 g/kg per day
Elderly	1.2 g/kg to 1.5g/kg per day

Preventing Malnutrition

Other specific interventions your loved one's physician and medical caregiving team may consider necessary include the following:

- Consulting with a dietician and others (speech therapist, physical therapist, for example) regarding changes in consistency of food
- Consulting with a pharmacist to discuss reducing or eliminating medications commonly implicated as risk factors for malnutrition
- Assessing and treating depression
- Conducting laboratory tests to detect underlying illnesses or conditions contributing to malnutrition
- Treating underlying infections, illnesses, or conditions causing malnutrition

- Implementing a bowel program for the elderly patient who is chronically constipated
- Beginning physical and/or occupational therapy or an exercise program. These will benefit those who need assistance building physical strength to allow self-feeding. Exercise will also stimulate healthy metabolism (called "anabolism") so that the body can begin to use nutrients properly again.
- Identifying, evaluating, and beginning therapy for those with dysphagia and other swallowing problems
- Providing supplemental feedings as required
- Tube feeding if ordered by the physician

If nutritional status is an issue with your loved one, the best way you can ensure recovery is either to be at the nursing home at mealtimes or to make sure someone is there to feed your loved one. You may consider hiring someone whose only job is to feed your loved one. The largest meal of the day is at noon, and as you will note when you visit, there are usually so many elders who need assistance with eating that it is difficult for nursing homes to provide the care needed.

In addition, there are some fairly easy techniques you can use to encourage your loved one to eat more calories and protein. You can:

ENCOURAGE AN INCREASE IN FLUIDS TO HELP IMPROVE NUTRITION

- Use ice chips, Popsicles, etc., as explained in the previous chapter to incorporate more liquids into her diet.
- Use wide, shallow glasses for drinking instead of tall, narrow ones. This will prevent air swallowing, which interferes with nutrition.
- Be careful not to wash food down with a liquid. This will lessen the danger of aspiration pneumonia.
- Encourage your loved one not to use straws for chewing and swallowing problems. Straws increase air swallowing and add to the number of steps required for drinking.
- Make sure your loved one has a ready and ample supply of fortified nutritional drinks such as Carnation Instant Breakfast ® or Ensure ® since these are a good source of nutrition. Some of these drinks have fiber, which is also important in your loved one's diet. Or you could use a powdered protein, available at health food stores, to make a high-protein drink.

INCREASE THE AMOUNT OF FOOD EATEN

- Feed your loved one small amounts of food first, then gradually increase the amount as her ability to swallow increases.
- Choose nutrient-dense foods such as eggs, dairy foods, and lean meats that provide high levels of protein and calories in small quantities of food.
- Serve your loved one several small meals instead of three large meals daily and offer snacks often.
- If your loved one is in a nursing home, suggest specific foods to the staff that you know are her favorites. In the alternative, bring her food from home, especially if you've made ethnic foods that she's always loved.
- Use herbs, seasonings, low-sodium beef, chicken, and vegetable flavors, lemon juice, orange juice, maple syrup, and bacon bits to boost the flavor of foods.
- Serve foods at appropriate temperatures. You can stimulate her appetite with warm or hot foods, which carry stronger smells.
- Choose foods that are not too challenging for your loved one to eat. Foods that have a double consistency such as anything with a skin (i.e., peas and grapes) may be difficult for her to manage.

ASSIST YOUR LOVED ONE IN EATING

- Use cueing techniques to encourage your loved one to eat. If she is not swallowing between spoonfuls, put an empty spoon into her mouth to trigger her swallowing mechanism. This technique is particularly helpful with cognitively impaired persons such as Alzheimer patients.
- Watch for aspiration. Never feed your loved one while she is lying down if at all possible, and do not tilt her head back. If she must be fed in bed, prop her up with pillows.
- If your loved one is dysphagic and is pocketing food (pushing food into the cheeks where it sits, partially chewed, without being swallowed), ask her speech therapist for assistance with safe feeding techniques. In particular, be aware that those with dysphagia need to sit upright at a 90-degree angle when eating to avoid aspiration of food and liquids.
- Use foods that stimulate your loved one's taste buds. This, plus your warm and loving presence, will encourage her continuing

interest in foods through the meal. If your loved one is in a nursing home, ask the staff where they keep such items as orange sherbet. Usually, this is freely available. The piquant taste of sherbet helps stimulate an interest in eating. This is also useful with those suffering from dementia.

USE ADAPTIVE MEASURES

- If your loved one has poor eyesight, use dishes that contrast with the tabletop.
- Make her forks and spoons easier to lift and hold by placing foam rubber hair curlers over the handles.

CONSIDER DIETARY SUPPLEMENTS

This intervention is controversial, but some physicians argue that use of a protein/calorie supplement doesn't have the desired effect. They say it doesn't result in an increase in total energy intake but rather in a decrease in habitual food intake and no significant change in total energy intake,[26] although one study showed that the use of supplements resulted in a small increase in body weight among nursing home residents.[27]

USE GROWTH HORMONES AND STEROIDS

Rarely are growth hormones and anabolic steroids used to increase appetite and body weight and/or muscle growth in the aged. If they are pre-scribed for your loved one, be sure to watch her closely for side effects. Although such drugs can increase appetite and promote weight gain, a large range of severe side effects, particularly affecting the aged, will make them appropriate only in selected geriatric patients.[28] Also, because these drugs are expensive, few elderly patients will likely be able to use them.

Tube Feeding

If your loved one suffers the effects of malnutrition, including PEM, her physicians might suggest using tube feeding. A primary concern for your loved one, yourself, and your other family members is that once tube feed-ing is started, it is very difficult to deal with the question of whether or when it should be discontinued. Tube feeding is a controversial topic for many reasons. The decision whether to begin tube feeding will depend upon several factors including medical status, mental status, and quality of life. In general, the following are indicators that tube feeding should be used:

- Your loved one suffers from a disease or condition that impairs swallowing such as Parkinson's disease or dysphagia.
- Your loved one has an increased metabolic rate. This might occur if she is recovering from surgery or an injury such as a broken hip. As stated earlier, anabolic (healthy) metabolism is needed to stimulate her production of tissue and she may likely be unable to meet her nutritional needs through eating alone.
- Your loved one suffers from a disease or condition such as cancer or malnutrition, but is otherwise mentally alert with a fair to good quality of life.
- Your loved one has an underlying condition that prevents her eating at this time, but she is expected to recover and continue a normal life. For example, she may be a postoperative patient or she may need the temporary use of a ventilator.

TYPES OF TUBE FEEDING

There are several different kinds of tube feeding. The type that your loved one's physician may recommend for her will depend entirely upon her particular health condition and her needs.

Total parenteral nutrition (TPN) or intravenous feeding. TPN is used to provide nutrients during a short-term recovery process. The nutrients are macronutrients in simplest form along with micronutrients (vitamins and minerals). This type of tube feeding provides all of the patient's daily nutritional requirements. The tube bypasses the stomach and nourishment is delivered directly into the bloodstream through a major vein. Your loved one could get sufficient nutrients with TPN to maintain weight indefinitely. TPN may be used to maintain nutritional status and to provide protein for building new tissue if your loved one is comatose or if she's had major surgery, multiple fractures, or severe burns, but is expected to survive. Since there are some serious complications of TPN such as blood clots and infection and because TPN is very expensive, your loved one's physician will not recommend it except in cases where it is absolutely indicated.

Nasogastric (NG) tube. A nasogastric (NG) tube, in which nutrients are supplied through an NG tube, is used for short-term tube feeding, for example in a post-operative stage of treatment. The NG tube is threaded into one nostril, down the throat and esophagus, and into the stomach. The tube is temporary and is uncomfortable for the patient. Because serious potential complications may arise, NG feeding is not often used.[29]

Percutaneous endoscopic gastrostomy (PEG). PEG is the most common type of tube feeding and arguably is the best route, because complications are not all that frequent. If your loved one needs PEG feeding, her physician can insert the PEG using only local anesthesia and intravenous (IV) sedation. The procedure is safe and usually takes about 20 to 40 minutes. The PEG feeding tube is inserted into the stomach directly through the abdominal wall. Feeding can begin with clear fluids between four and 24 hours after the procedure, which may be done on an outpatient basis. The patient may return to her own home or to a nursing home following the procedure. A PEG can be used for temporary feedings or can be permanent. A PEG will last for months. [30]

A decision to institute PEG feedings should not be made lightly. PEG is appropriate for patients who have an intact, functional gastrointestinal tract but are unable, because of a disease or condition, to consume sufficient calories to meet metabolic needs. Common reasons for PEG feedings are neurologic disorders such as Alzheimer's or Parkinson's disease or severe stroke associated with difficulty in swallowing. Obstructions such as cancerous growths in the throat, larynx, or esophagus are another reason why PEG feedings might be considered. PEG is not appropriate in patients whose incurable disease is progressing rapidly. NG feedings over a short period can produce the same result.

DECIDING WHETHER TUBE FEEDING IS APPROPRIATE FOR YOUR LOVED ONE

When you and your loved one, if she can participate, consider whether she should have tube feeding, explore the following issues with her doctor:

- The reason for placement of a tube
- The possible adverse events
- The likelihood that an adverse event will occur
- The expected outcome of tube feeding (the benefits)
- The expectations about length of therapy

It may be beneficial for your loved one's normal oral intake of food to be supplemented using PEG feeding on a short-term basis, particularly if she's just been discharged from the hospital after a stroke, surgery, or illness. PEG feeding can provide her with the extra protein that is essential to healthy wound healing and can be useful in helping her recover. Another plus to consider is this: feeding through a PEG tube can be given during the night, so she can eat normally during the day and can also take part in physical therapy and social activities.[31] Thus tube feeding can help her avoid or overcome malnutrition, but she may still enjoy the social and emotional aspects of normal daily living,

The results of various studies exploring whether there is any benefit at all for elderly patients to have tube feeding conflict. Some studies show that there is no improvement in the quality of life and that it doesn't prolong survival. Other studies associate tube feeding with better wound healing and a lower rate of late mortality.

Dr. Morley states that tube feeding is not a universal remedy and that few nursing home residents benefit from it. In commenting on his research, he says that the lack of good results might be explained by the relatively poor status of a nursing home resident at the time tube feeding is initiated. Still, he cautions that for many nursing home residents, tube feeding merely prolongs life and does not provide quality of life. He believes the decision of whether to tube feed patients depends as much on what the patients and their families want as it does on medical necessity. Often, he says, a decision to tube feed is made on an emergency basis without consideration for whether the feeding will improve life or merely prolong it.[32]

What it really boils down to are the wishes and values of your loved one and your family. It's not possible to predict the long-term effects feeding tubes have on survival. What one person will find acceptable in terms of quality of life may be very intolerable to another. The decision to initiate tube feeding should be carefully made, weighing the negative aspects against potential benefits. You and your loved one should know there is a choice in the matter. (See Chapter Nine for this discussion.) Usually, that choice will center on what your loved one's quality of life is, what the benefits to prolonging her life are, and what her wishes for end-of-life care are.

CHAPTER EIGHT

Understaffing: A Threat in Those Nursing Homes

NOVEMBER, 2000

Although I filed the petition to be Mom's guardian in early November, prior to the time we moved Mom to Traverse City, establishing a guardianship can take more than a month. This can have dire consequences for patients.

Mom was transferred from Alpine Manor to the Traverse City nursing home on November 8, and I was soon informed that they would be unable to use the side rails of the bed more than another day without agreement from a court-appointed guardian. State investigations into nursing home resident deaths as a result of strangulation after being caught in the bedrails had made nursing homes wary about liability issues. Only if a legal guardian signed a waiver of liability would the nursing home agree to use the bedrails after a very brief period.

Because Mom's condition was so unstable in the days just after her transfer to Traverse City and her safety was an issue, I filed an amended petition with the court asking for an emergency order appointing me as Mom's temporary guardian. The court appointed a guardian ad litem for Mom, a lawyer who visited Mom in the nursing home that same day and advised the court as to her condition. The guardian ad litem recommended the appointment and an order was entered within 24 hours naming me as her temporary guardian. Consequently, we were able to use the side rails of the bed. We were lucky. This is not the norm, and in counties that are larger than Grand Traverse County, where caseloads may be heavier, delays are common.

Mom's first week in the Traverse City facility flew by. I typically arrived at the nursing home by 10:00 a.m., with plenty of time to talk with the staff and also to feed Mom lunch at noon. Each day was occupied with an assessment of Mom's diet, medical and health status, and motor capabilities. The first day, the director of nursing and others were at Mom's side during lunch. They noted that she was not able to eat a mechanical soft diet, as Alpine Manor had stated on her discharge summary. Mom's diet was accordingly switched to an intermediate processed food diet and, on the third day, to a puréed diet. The nursing home's dietician, occupational, physical, and speech therapists also participated in the assessment. As it became apparent that Mom would need to be fed at each meal, I made it known that I would be there to feed her as often as possible and certainly at noon, which was her big meal of the day.

The staff was encouraging and helpful. Each day they spent the entire hour that it took to feed Mom with us, explaining to me the difficulties Mom was having with swallowing, how she tended to pocket food in her left cheek, the dangers of aspiration, and the techniques, such as cueing, that would facilitate feeding Mom. The director of nursing showed me Mom's chart and explained to me that she was "at risk" for malnutrition. I now know that if we had used BMI to assess her, her BMI of 18 would have triggered a full alert and attempts to reverse what was by then an irreversible negative process. Mom's chart did not, however, note her as "at risk" for dehydration.

The staff showed me the pantry where they kept liquid supplements and orange sherbet used to stimulate the taste buds and encourage eating. I was told to help myself whenever I thought Mom needed anything. I bought the "sippy cups" young children use for Mom's liquids as it was apparent that she could not sip through a straw and that drinking was very difficult for her. I made signs for her door and also for the room that invited anyone in the room to help Mom with a drink of water if she were alert and sitting up. I worried that I was not there after 6:00 p.m., from after dinner through the night. Who would make sure Mom had liquids during this time?

Each day the staff spent a considerable amount of time trying to determine how to help Mom sit comfortably and safely in her wheelchair. Looking back, I recall that staying in the chair was really a problem for Mom. Her body sometimes was rigid. Sometimes uncontrollable tremors threatened to catapult her from the chair. Now I know that these were signs of neurological damage that should have triggered admission to the hospital and the complete neurological assessment that Dr. Belle had suggested. One of the problems, of course, was that the staff did not know what was normal for Mom. It was difficult for them to see the rigidity and tremors as abnormal. It was also difficult for them to sort out the parkinsonism that was an EPS from tremors related to her Parkinson's disease.

The tremors increased in strength on Thursday, two days after we'd transferred Mom. These were involuntary and not like the tremors I'd seen in Alpine Manor. Instead, Mom's whole body rocked with exaggerated spasms, making it difficult for her to sit in her wheelchair. I called these to the attention of the director of nursing and other staff members. Mom's new physician had not yet been *in to see her, and I'd hand-delivered a summary of what I thought her condition was to his office with a note asking him to see her as soon as possible.*

After her meal, Mom lay down for a nap and I spent over an hour at the nurses' station reviewing her medical records. That was when I noted that Alpine Manor had precipitously eliminated the antipsychotic medication just before her transfer. I didn't know much about psychoactive drugs, but I thought immediately of withdrawal symptoms as a cause for her tremors and brought this to the attention of the director of nursing. She examined Mom and then telephoned the physician's office. He prescribed Benadryl for her and then came to the nursing home in the early evening. He did not perceive a need to transfer her to the hospital, but he did order neurological testing to be done the following week.

Jill and her daughter, Allison, arrived on Saturday to see Mom. Both were shocked at her appearance. As the weekend progressed, I had my first experience with what nursing home staffing is like on weekends. During the week, there had been much assistance and evaluation. But on the weekend, there were strange and inexperienced aides. Two aides who were supposed to transfer Mom from her wheelchair to her bed after a meal seemed to be completely inexperienced and nearly dropped her. Just as they got her into her bed, Mom expelled everything she'd eaten in an incident of abrupt, uncontrollable diarrhea. The aides shook their heads in disgust and left, not coming back to attend to her until I went to the desk and expressed concern. As Mom continued to have uncontrollable tremors and to be unable to sit in her chair, I asked the staff to leave her in bed for her meal on Sunday. Looking back, I should have had them call the physician. I simply failed to understand how critical Mom's condition was. By this point, Mom's stomach was unable to absorb nutrition as a result of what none of us understood—that she had already suffered massive damage due to dehydration and malnutrition.

The Serious Problem of Understaffing

According to the most recent federal study, as of 2000, over 91% of the nursing homes in this country have insufficient nurse aide staffing levels to provide the necessary care to nursing home residents. Over 40% of these nursing homes would have to increase nurse aide staff by 50% or more to reach the minimum threshold necessary to meet the residents' needs.[1]

How can this be when federal laws supposedly regulate nursing homes and the level of staffing in nursing homes? The laws are inadequate to begin with, they are not routinely enforced, and they are simply insufficient to protect your loved one from dire consequences. This will be particularly true if she is seriously debilitated, delirious, or suffering from dementia and thus unable to properly access liquids and food.

There is a direct correlation between higher staffing levels in nursing homes and good outcomes for residents. The benefits of higher staffing include lower mortality rates, improved physical functioning, fewer decubitus ulcers (bedsores), fewer catheterized residents, lower rates of urinary tract infections, and a decreased use of antibiotics.

On the other hand, serious medical consequences commonly arise in nursing homes as a result of staffing levels that are too low. In fact, inadequate staffing and inadequately trained staff contribute to poor nutritional intake, undiagnosed dysphagia, poor oral health, resident deterioration, hospitalization, malnutrition, dehydration, and starvation.[2]

Here are the facts. Residents receive an average of 42 minutes of care per day from RNs (including the director of nursing) and an average of 42 minutes from LPN/LVNs. Some of those minutes of care include all direct-care activities, but more of their time is spent on indirect tasks, such as administration, charting, measuring out and distributing medication doses, and staff breaks. On average, each competency evaluated nurse assistant (CENA) delivers care for 12 residents and each RN or LPN usually supervises care for 32 to 34 residents during their 8-hour shifts. 60% of the total care—126 minutes per resident per day—is given by CENAs, who are required to have minimal training and who receive low wages and benefits.

It is well-documented in a 1998 report issued by the Health Care Financing Administration (HCFA) that in more than half—54%—of the nursing homes surveyed, nursing aides spent *less than two hours a day with patients.* The report also said the elderly involved were at great risk for dehydration.[3]

Even more shocking is a 1997 report showing that physicians (the medical director, the attending physician, and physician extenders, such as nurse practitioners) *spent an average of only one minute per resident per day in nursing facilities.*[4]

Federal laws and regulations mandate that a nursing home resident be seen by her assigned physician at least once a month, more often if the nursing staff alerts her to complications. But having regulations and laws on the books isn't, in and of itself, enough to protect your loved one. After all, in the five weeks that Mom was in the skilled nursing and the long-term care section of Alpine Manor, her assigned doctor *never* saw her!

It simply didn't occur to me or to my sisters that our mother was receiving only an average of 3.5 hours of direct *and* indirect care from all sources in a 24-hour period.[5] We did not realize that there was really very little actual "hands-on" evaluative nursing care. Nor did we realize that most of the care nursing home residents receive is given by persons who have less training than we'd have expected our childcare givers to have!

It's going to be up to you to make sure that these facts do not prove fatal to your loved one during her nursing home stay. The incidence of understaffing is higher than you might possibly imagine, making it imperative that you carefully monitor your loved one's care and condition.

Nursing Homes Are Seriously Understaffed

Over 91% of the nursing homes in this country have insufficient nurse aide staffing levels to provide the necessary care. Over 40% of all nursing homes would have to increase nurse aide staff by 50% or more to reach the minimum threshold necessary.

You don't need to know all the horrifying facts about how serious this problem is, but if your loved one is going to spend any time in a nursing home, no matter what the reputation of that facility, you will want to read the definitive report on nursing home deficiencies, including understaffing, so that you can protect your loved one from injury or death. You can read this online or you can download it to your computer. See Burger, SJ, Kayser-Jones J, Prince J. Malnutrition and dehydration in nursing homes: Key issues in prevention and treatment. Commonwealth Fund. 2000 July; Pub. No. 386. This report can be found at www.nccnhr.org/pdf/burger_mal_386.pdf.

Facilities that are certified for Medicare only (skilled care) have the highest staffing levels.[6] Unfortunately, most nursing home care is paid for by Medicaid; Medicare does not pay for nursing home care beyond a brief period of recuperation after a hospitalization. Thus, few elderly persons in nursing facilities will experience nursing home care offering such generous care.

Contact with Physicians

In 1997, a report showed that physicians spent an average of one minute per resident day in nursing facilities—meaning 30 minutes per month per resident.

According to Burger's 2000 report, the following factors are common to most nursing homes and contribute to the decline of the residents of those nursing homes: a failure to individualize care to each resident's needs, inadequate staffing, high turnover among nurses' aides, and a failure of trained professionals to supervise the aides.

Burger gave an example of how the lack of education and continuing education can contribute to malnutrition and dehydration of residents: when questioned about what they remembered learning regarding feeding techniques in their training, the CENAs in one study merely remembered being taught "how to calculate the percentage of food eaten, that the head of the bed should be elevated, and that they should sit down when feeding residents."[7]

Those residents most at risk are those who lack of family or friends to assist them at mealtimes, especially those with moderate to severe dysphagia, those who have severe mental and functional impairment, those who have aphasia (loss of the ability to speak due to injury or disease in the brain), and those who don't speak English.[8]

Burger voiced similar concerns about the lack of supervision of CENAs by the nursing staff. This is particularly important in the resident with dysphagia, for example, who must be fed carefully to avoid aspiration of food or liquids. Burger's report that cited the prevalence of protein/energy malnutrition reviewed in Chapter Seven linked PEM—its cause or its exacerbation—to the fact that many, if not most, U.S. nursing homes are understaffed. There simply aren't enough aides to give enough care to the residents, particularly at mealtimes.

Making matters worse is the fact that nursing homes often hire contract workers to fill in as there never seem to be enough CENAs. A study cited by Burger established a 93.3% per year turnover rate for CENAs! One can understand such a rate when you consider that these jobs are very difficult and, typically, not very rewarding. The work is hard; it often is dirty and unpleasant. It also pays poorly—usually minimum wage or a few dollars more per hour.

But just imagine how much higher the risk of dehydration or malnutrition is for the elderly resident who is cared for by an aide who is new or by a contract worker filling in where CENAs have quit. It is here that the lack of continuity of care I earlier cited as a major danger for your loved one becomes critical. Even with a care plan, a newly hired CENA or a temporary contract worker may not know how to care for a resident already at risk for malnutrition and dehydration.

In addition, *having* a care plan is not the same thing as *following* a care plan. According to Burger, a lack of supervisory licensed nurses, as well as their lack of nutritional knowledge, leaves CENAs to do the best they can without appropriate help from professionals.

Although Burger suggests ways that nursing homes should address these problems, family caregivers should be aware that little has been accomplished since Burger's report was published. Unless your loved one is in a most unique facility, it will be up to you to monitor her care and even assist with her care, if you possibly can do so. Look around the dining area at your loved one's facility. How many staff persons are assisting at the semicircular table reserved for those residents who need help eating and drinking? When Burger's report was written, it was typical for one staff person to be assigned to seven to nine residents during the daytime meal and 12 to 15 during the evening meal. Residents fed in such circumstances only have about six minutes with an aide at each meal, which is not enough time for them to be fed adequately and sufficiently. This becomes critical if your loved one has difficulty swallowing and requires a long time to feed safely and sufficiently, usually an hour.

Because staffing levels are usually inadequate to meet the needs of the large numbers of nursing home residents who require assistance at mealtimes, you should carefully evaluate the care available to your loved one. Are there others assisting at mealtimes such as administrators or indirect care workers? Are there family members and volunteers to assist with feeding and socializing?

In order that you appreciate the danger to your loved one, consider the following anecdotal evidence cited by Burger that suggests malnutrition and dehydration also occur in facilities *with* adequate numbers of staff, because of the lack of appropriate management and supervision. In 1999, an ombudsmen group observed meals in 80 nursing homes, both during the week and on weekends. Burger's quotes from their unpublished report are shocking:[9]

- I observed several people playing with their food, not really eating. No one came over to help or to give encouragement. They just took the trays away.
- Staff attitude is bad. They act like it is a great inconvenience that they have to help anybody.
- A resident said she sometimes missed meals because they forgot her.
- I watched a man trying to feed himself breakfast. He had spilled his milk and coffee. The toast was on the floor. He was trying to

eat cold cereal and milk with a spoon but most of it never reached his mouth. After about 15 minutes he just gave up. There was an aide sitting in the day room with him. She was reading the paper and never even looked up.

- No water was served with the meal.
- The administrator informed me that they are not required to monitor food consumption.
- I observed CENAs charting food consumption without actually looking at the trays.

The amount of time spent with each resident by professionals directly correlates to risk of malnutrition and dehydration for the resident. The good *and* bad news is that all the professionals who come into contact with residents can contribute to their well-being, or lack of it. Physicians can affect the nutritional status of residents because they can detect risks that predispose a resident to malnutrition or dehydration. They can also order and interpret diagnostics to help detect changes in status affecting nutrition and hydration. But a doctor who sees a patient once a month is unlikely to detect changes in status early enough to order preventative measures.

Similarly, nurses are responsible for directing the care of residents by delegating CENAs to assist affected residents. Nurses, who have so much more contact with residents than physicians, must also monitor the nutritional status of residents and make referrals to a dietician or to a speech therapist for evaluation of swallowing disorders. But according to Burger's research, registered dieticians, who are trained to assess each resident's fluid and nutrition needs and who can direct how these needs should be met, are usually only present in a nursing home 3.3 hours per week.[10] Research shows this to be insufficient.

How You Can Minimize the Effects of Understaffing for Your Loved One

When I first began writing this book, it was my opinion that, if possible, loved ones should be kept at home rather than placed in a nursing home. One of my friends said, "Easy for you to say! What you propose is not practical for most people."

I agree. Even though keeping loved ones at home is preferable, in many cases it simply will not work. This is particularly true in the case of patients with degenerative diseases like Alzheimer's. Even so, my later research proved that the majority of the frail elderly, about 80%, do live in the community.[11]

In part, this is because nursing home care is expensive: it costs $40,000 per year or more. Some people have long-term care insurance, but amazingly, 52 million Americans provide "informal care" to a family member or friend who is disabled or ill. That's one out of every three adults between the ages of 20 and 75! Though some of this care is provided to seniors who live in assisted living facilities or in nursing homes, most is provided at home. The Department of Disability, Aging, and Long-Term Care Policy calls this "Compassion in Action."[12]

Whatever your choice for a care setting, your loved one will probably spend some time, perhaps a brief recuperation after surgery or a major illness, in a nursing home. This is not necessarily a bad thing, and you can help your loved one make the best of it. There are five main ways you can do so: investigate deficiencies, place quality of care ahead of location, monitor your loved one's care, assist at meals, and consider hiring a geriatric care manager.

INVESTIGATE DEFICIENCIES

An important consideration in selecting a facility is the number of deficiencies the facility has received and the scope and severity of those deficiencies. Federal and state standards regarding resident care and safety must be met to receive a state license and/or federal certification. Inspectors from each state's department of health services licensing and certification program survey nursing homes every 12 to15 months to determine whether minimum standards are being met.[13]

The federal government has 185 such quality standards, and each state has many additional standards of care and safety that facilities must meet. When a nursing facility does not comply with a standard (or regulation), it is issued a deficiency citation. Nursing homes may also receive a deficiency in response to authenticated complaints from residents or other interested persons. Deficiencies are grouped into one of eight distinct categories on the Nursing Home Compare Website: quality of care, abuse, resident assessment, resident rights, environment, nutrition, pharmacy, and administration.

Nursing Home Deficiencies

Deficiencies are an indication of the quality of care provided by a facility. Don't look only at the number of deficiencies. Look at the scope and severity of deficiencies and whether they are corrected or repeated.

Deficiencies are an indication of the quality of care provided by the facility, but it is not merely the number of deficiencies that matters, it is the scope and severity and whether a repeated pattern of deficiencies occurs. This information may be easily retrieved from the Medicare Nursing Home Compare website at www.hcfa.gov/medicare.[14] Recurring violations of the same type and a high number of serious violations are the most important indicators of quality. Sadly, although I checked with a state ombudsman about the quality of care in Traverse City, I failed to appreciate the significance of what they told me. They said that the facility I'd chosen had been cited for not making water readily available. Because of my lack of knowledge and experience, I did not appreciate the level of risk this presented for Mom. I encourage you not to be so complacent.

See www.nccnhr.org/static_pages/ombudsmen_list.cfm for the name and contact information for your state ombudsman. This individual will be able to tell you of the violations or citations a specific nursing home has had. Later, after placement, if problems arise that you are unable to resolve with the administration, the ombudsman is available to assist you.

If placement is to be in an adult foster care home, a state agency can assist you in narrowing down the choices. A placement consultant can direct you to facilities with resident populations compatible with the interests and abilities of your loved one. The consultant can also provide you with a list and description of any citations or violations of the AFCH. Michigan's state agency is called the Family Independence Agency. In other states, you will undoubtedly find an agency on aging that can direct you to the appropriate office.

PLACE QUALITY OF CARE AHEAD OF LOCATION

Families usually select a nursing facility based on geographic location— that is, whether the facility is located near their loved one's home or the home of relatives or friends. Cost may be a consideration, but often little thought is given to the quality of care. This may be particularly true when there is little time in which to choose a facility. But the quality of care can vary widely across facilities. Location is not the best reason for selecting a facility. Your primary consideration should be high quality of care.

If you have access to the Internet, there is a resource available to assist you in evaluating nursing facilities based upon quality of care. A nursing home information system was established on the Internet in 1999 by the Centers for Medicare and Medicaid Services (CMS), formerly the Health Care Financing Administration.

This website provides comparison data from the federal surveys of all 16,500 nursing facilities in the United States that are certified to provide Medicare and Medicaid services. It provides basic information about facilities (location, bed size, occupancy) as well as information about the residents who live at the nursing home (percent with pressure sores and other conditions), about nurse staffing, and also about deficiencies. The website is interactive, and users can select three facilities at a time in an area for comparison purposes. About 100,000 individuals per month use this website as a valuable resource. It may be accessed at www.Medicare. gov/NursingHomeCompare.htm.

One of the most important factors to consider in selecting a nursing home is whether the facility has adequate nursing staff to provide high quality of care. In short, consumers should look for facilities that have the highest possible staffing levels. Research shows that nursing facilities that are hospital-based as well as non-profit facilities generally have higher staffing levels, and higher staffing usually means better quality of care.

MONITOR YOUR LOVED ONE'S CARE

Should you choose a nursing facility for your loved one, you can't just drop her off and go on about your life while depending on the facility or physician to make sure proper care is given. Under the best of circumstances, there are just too many things that can go wrong that, in a matter of hours or days, can cause an elderly person to die. When holidays or weekends intervene, even hospitals are short-staffed. Further, the staff on duty is not always the most experienced. The only way to protect your loved one is to consistently monitor the care she receives. This includes everything from the medications she is given to the amount of food she consumes to her behaviors. Our family thought Alpine Manor's staff was professional and trained to care for Mom. We were grievously mistaken, and Mom died because of it.

ASSIST AT MEALS

Residents who have family members to assist with eating are unlikely to lose weight.[15] Therefore, you can help the most by assisting your loved one with eating, especially at the noontime meal, which is the main meal in nursing homes. It is important to have training from the nursing staff in techniques that will best meet the special challenges your loved one presents; be sure to find out which professionals are appropriate to teach you these feeding techniques. Typically, these will be speech, occupational, or physical therapists.

Also, since your loved one's status depends in part on the accuracy of her nutrition and liquid intake report, if you decide to help at mealtimes, be sure to find out to whom to report her intake so that her records are accurate. In particular, if you become aware that your loved one's intake has changed, be sure to discuss this not only with the aide but also with her nurse or the director of nursing. Make sure you also report changes in function or any new symptoms that will impair her ability to take in nutrients or fluids. Get to know the people who are responsible for your loved one's care. Make sure they know when you arrive and when you leave. If you'll be away for a period of days, be sure to let the appropriate people know so that your loved one isn't, in effect, abandoned if you don't show up.

CONSIDER HIRING A GERIATRIC CARE MANAGER

If you live far away from the nursing home where your loved one resides, consider hiring a geriatric care manager to oversee her medical, physical, and legal status. A geriatric care manager is a professional trained in gerontology, social work, nursing, and/or counseling who may visit with the elderly, evaluate and monitor their situation, and arrange medical and other appointments. Such a person may act as a liaison for your family to ensure that your loved one's needs are met. See Appendix F for more details.

In these ways, you can take charge of monitoring your loved one's medical, physical, and cognitive status. If you decide to do this, you will surely add years to her life as well as to the quality of her life. Because of the inadequacy of the limited care provided in nursing homes, the best person to monitor your loved ones' status is you.

CHAPTER NINE

Facing End-of-Life Issues and Making Choices

NOVEMBER 13, 2000

I arrived at the nursing home shortly before 10:30 a.m. and was surprised to be met at once by the director of nursing. She said, "Jeanne, we left a message on your answering machine. We've not been able to awaken your mom. We think perhaps she should be taken to the hospital."

I agreed to go alone to Mom's room to see her and to make a decision. It was soon clear to me that I could not rouse her, so I returned to the front desk and gave the okay to call the ambulance.

Everything that followed that day remains a blur. The ambulance arrived and Mom was prepared for transfer. At some point, I was handed Mom's glasses, which I stuck in my jacket pocket. Many months later when I found them, I would turn them over and over in my hand, bewildered about whose they were, and then, stunned when the realization hit me, say to Glen, "These are Mommy's glasses."

I arrived in the emergency room just after the ambulance had arrived. The staff led me into a room where Mom was lying on an examining table. Her eyes were closed and her breathing was rapid but shallow. Soon, Dr. John arrived. Then Glen came in.

For a long time afterwards, I wondered how Glen had known Mom was in the hospital. I'd forgotten that he had planned to meet me at the nursing home so we could discuss a modification of Mom's wheelchair to make her more comfortable. Of course, the director of nursing had told him to come to the hospital.

People came and went from Mom's side; blood samples were drawn as assessments were made. Finally Dr. John came in and told us that Mom was in "multisystem failure." He said that she would be taken to a room soon and he would begin a full battery of neurological tests. He gave me the name of a neurologist who would consult with him.

It was nearly 2:00 p.m. by the time Mom was transferred to a room. She was in a double and her roommate was watching one TV program after another. The din was quite awful. I drew the curtains around Mom's bed and kept the lights dimmed. People came and went, drawing more samples, fitting Mom with an oxygen mask and then monitoring it every hour, and turning Mom.

In the late afternoon, a hospital staff member—a phlebotomist—came in.[1] She and Mom's nurse discussed changing the shunt to Mom's IV. As I sat by Mom's bedside, I could hear her concern as she was unable to get Mom to relax her arm so that the shunt could be changed.

"I can help you," I said. I stepped to Mom's side and took her left hand. Her arm was rigidly clenched, and when I tried to lower her hand to the bed, she seemed to pull it back toward her shoulder. I know now that this was "cog-wheel rigidity," a sign of a neurological condition and, in fact, one of the presenting symptoms for neuroleptic malignant syndrome. But at the time, I found her rigidity only odd and unnatural.

"Mom, it's Jeannie," I said. As I spoke, I lightly ran my fingernails up and down the inside of her forearm. "There's a nurse here who is going to change your IV so it isn't so uncomfortable." I continued to lightly stroke her as her arm relaxed, and I lowered it to the bed. Carefully, I kept my left hand on hers and put my right hand just above her elbow, making sure that when the IV was being changed, Mom would not jerk her arm away and get hurt. I lay my upper body down next to hers, putting my head near hers on the pillow. Closing my eyes, I began to tell Mom a story to distract her from the procedure. While Mom appeared unconscious, I espouse the theory that all people, whether conscious or not, can hear everything said around them. It seemed important then and later that Mom have continuing assurance that I was at her bedside.

"Mom, do you remember when we lived on Adams Street?" I began. "There was just Kay, Betsy, and me then. We lived in a little white house on the corner, not far from Grandma's house. Do you remember the little sailor dresses that Grandma Parkin sewed for us? We got all dressed up and went to the train station to meet Daddy's train when he came home from the war. We waved flags and sang "God Bless America," or was it "Bell Bottom Trousers?" I remember that we greeted him with hugs and tears. Do you remember that?

"Mom, do you remember the train that went by our house every day? Kay and I used to stand out by the tracks to watch it. The engineer threw coal out of the big steam engine that we would use to draw pictures on the sidewalk. When we were little, we thought he was throwing the coal to us. Now I realize he was throwing it at us, trying to discourage us from standing so close to the tracks."
I continued. "Mom, do you remember the day Kay and I went to visit Grandma on the other side of the railroad tracks? Grandma wasn't home and we wanted

some cookies. So we took her kitchen sheers and cut a huge bouquet of flowers from her garden and left it for her on the kitchen table with the cookie crumbs!" Mom lay unmoving and finally I opened my eyes to find that her IV had been successfully changed. Mom was so quiet. What would this day bring?

November 13–20, 2000

Phone calls were made to alert Betsy and Jill that Mom was in the hospital. Although I left the hospital in the early evening, I was there by 9:00 or 10:00 a.m. each day. Mom was supported by IVs containing glucose, nutrients to correct her electrolyte imbalance, a diuretic to combat the congestive heart failure and edema, and also a powerful antibiotic. Each day diagnostic tests ordered by Mom's physicians were done. Each day I awaited the early evening visits by the physicians. Both the internist and the neurologist remained puzzled about what had precipitated this crisis. Of course, lack of a good history was a very serious impediment to solving the problem. Because the disease that ultimately killed Mom is so rare, because these two physicians had no experience with Mom in the days when she was well, and because there was no adequate history, this particular disease was never considered as a diagnosis. Even today, I remain certain that it was impossible, under the circumstances, to diagnose. I am also sure that even had it been diagnosed, Mom's condition was so dire that we never could have saved her.

On Wednesday, Mom's nurse asked me if I were certain Mom was allergic to codeine. Her records indicated she was, but the nurse said it was very common for people to say they were allergic to codeine and other medications. Unless they'd experienced a rash when using codeine, however, they were not really allergic. Having an upset stomach because codeine was taken without food was a common cause of discomfort, but that did not amount to an allergy. It was important, she said, to determine whether there was really an allergy because Mom could not be given morphine, which she needed, if she were really allergic to codeine, an opiod (painkiller) in the same class of drugs. Much, much later, after Mom's death, I realized that Dr. John had decided it was time to give "comfort care."

I telephoned Glen and asked him to call Jill at work and have her call the hospital. Mom's nurse talked with Jill, asking her lots of questions, and finally decided that Mom probably was not allergic to morphine. At that moment, Dr. John appeared. While he was in the room, the nurse gave Mom a small amount of morphine. Both of them observed her until they were certain she was not going to have a reaction. Morphine became a friend and ally in those last days, allowing Mom to relax, to breathe more normally, and to feel no pain.

I had telephoned Kris, Mom's eldest grandson, to let him know his Nana was *critically ill. She was not, I told him, unaware of what was going on around her, but she was generally non-responsive and had not opened her eyes since her admission. I suggested that he telephone her to talk with her in mid-afternoon. Both Kris and his younger sister, Trisha, telephoned Nana on Tuesday. On Wednesday, Kris planned to telephone Mom at 6:30 p.m. The telephone rang just as the neurologist came in on her rounds. I asked Kris to call back and turned my attention to the neurologist's questions and suggestions.*

After she left, I said, "Mom that was Kris on the telephone. He's going to telephone you in about 15 minutes." I was certainly surprised when, as the telephone began to ring a half hour later (Kris had gotten busy), Mom sat upright in bed, opened her eyes, and turned her head toward the phone. I jumped from my seat, went to her side, answered the telephone, and asked Kris to hold on for a minute. Gently, I stroked Mom's shoulders and encouraged her to lie back down. When I got her settled onto her pillow, I held the receiver to her ear. I could hear Kris' voice talking to Mom very gently and soothingly.

It was amazing to see how Mom's face relaxed, how the furrows in her brows smoothed, how her forearms relaxed. She almost smiled as she lay there, eyes closed, listening to Kris' voice. When I heard Kris fall silent, I finally removed the receiver and spoke briefly to him with the report for the day. Basically, we didn't know any more than we had on Monday.

Friday was a very long day. Mom was scheduled to have an MRI mid-morning to determine whether a cerebral event was the cause of the acute failure of her kidney, neurological, and cardiopulmonary systems. She was still experiencing tremors and her nurse, Bill, was worried about whether she could lie still enough for a good "picture." Another nurse covered Bill's patients that morning while Bill worked with morphine and a mild anti-anxiety medication to eliminate the tremors as much as possible. The MRI was postponed, pending a lessening in the tremors, and finally around noon, Bill decided Mom was calm enough to justify the MRI. He called over to the MRI unit and a young man soon appeared in the doorway with a gurney. Mom was transferred to the gurney, the portable oxygen was hooked up, and we were off. Because Mom might need morphine before she went into the MRI machine, Bill had a syringe of morphine in one hand.

First we rolled past a utility room, and Bill grabbed three heated blankets from a warmer on the fly. Mom was covered with warm blankets and we rolled through halls, through a tunnel under the street, across an open alley, and into the freestanding building near the hospital where the MRI machine is kept. Bill monitored Mom every step of the way and, sure enough, his forethought about the morphine proved fortuitous. It was because of his determination and hard work that Mom was able to get a good quality MRI. As it turned out, the test itself was not determinative, except that it ruled out any cerebral-vascular event.

It was 7:00 p.m., snowing lightly, when I left the hospital. After a late dinner, Glen and I sat watching television. Suddenly, the telephone rang. It was Mom's nurse; she said Mom was having a rough night and suggested I come to the hospital. Quickly pulling on my parka, I drove through the snowy country-side toward the hospital. We live about 20 miles away and the roads are two-lane and winding. Coming down one of the more treacherous hills, I felt the car fish-tail dangerously. Recovering from the skid, I slowed down for the last eight miles. It was a very scary ride to town. Parking near the emergency room entrance, I went into the hospital and to Mom's room, arriving at about 10:00 p.m.

The nurses were wonderful, bringing me a reclining chair, pillows, blankets, and coffee. As I sat by Mom's bedside, I wondered what her nurse had meant by the statement that Mom was having a rough night. So far, she looked just as she had all day. At about 11:00 p.m., two nurses came in to turn Mom; turning took place every second hour to avoid bedsores. Within a half hour, I was roused from my drowsiness by a sound. Opening my eyes, I saw Mom sitting upright in bed, her eyes wide and her face contorted with fear. I rushed to her side, trying to assess the situation. Mom was having trouble breathing and she was terrified. I rang for the nurses, while I held Mom in my arms, trying to calm her.

When the nurses came, they quickly administered morphine and an anti-anxiety medication, injecting both into a port that was part of Mom's IV appa-ratus. I remained at her side for a long time, stroking her shoulders and arms, soothing her in a low voice. For the remainder of the evening I half slept in the chair, and each time the nurses came in to turn Mom and administer her med-ications, I would observe. Finally, I suggested that it was the turning that was raising Mom's level of consciousness and precipitating the respiratory crisis. "Couldn't we schedule the turning to occur one half hour after the morphine and anti-anxiety medications?" I asked.

There was rapid agreement. To ensure that other shifts would also do this, I wrote a note and taped it to the wall above Mom's head. I didn't know then that the nurses all met in a conference room between shifts with the staff coming on duty and that this resolution of the respiratory distress would be shared. And even though I believed that the nurses would handle Mom carefully, I slept little, keeping watch over her through the night.

On Saturday, groggy from little sleep, I was in the hallway talking to Dr. John when Jill arrived. He told us that none of the battery of neurological assessments had revealed any cause for Mom's condition. He explained that the MRI had been normal. There were only two other tests that could be ordered, a spinal tap to check for infectious processes such as meningitis, and a brain biopsy.

Jill and I said those procedures sounded too invasive and well beyond the scope of Mom's wishes as expressed in her patient advocacy designation. Also, we thought that even if the tests showed anything, Mom's condition was so marginal that there would be any way to cure her. Dr. John said he thought this was probably the case and that he did not really recommend going further. He felt that even if we lengthened her life by a small amount of time, her quality of life would be terrible.

I was finally beginning to accept the fact that Mom was not going to get better. Though I'd spoken with hospice on Friday and had arranged that Mom would come to our home as a hospice patient as soon as possible, just days earlier I'd arranged for the nursing home to hold her bed for that week, expecting that she would recover and go back to the nursing home.

Logistically, it was not possible to bring Mom home until Tuesday. We had to give the company that supplied the bed and oxygen time to make the delivery and to run the training session.

Monday, November 20, was spent caring for Mom and talking to hospice workers. Social workers came to Mom's bedside and one of them stood on the opposite side of the bed from me. In retrospect, I think she was probably sent to assess whether I could handle hospice work.

She asked me what I was doing for Mom and I replied that I'd been telling her stories about growing up and singing songs to her. She suggested that I stroke Mom, and I replied that I was trying very hard to respect Mom's sensitivities. Mom hadn't, I said, really liked to be touched. Talking with her, I said, was a good way of letting her know that I was by her side. I felt that it was also a good way of affirming Mom's worth as a mother and of giving her permission to leave.

I was determined, if death were to be the outcome of this crisis, to take Mom home and care for her until her death. I'd had a little exposure to hospice care, and it was comforting to think of Mom being with us at home where it would be quiet, where we could play soft music on the stereo, where we could keep the lights dimmed all the time, and where there would be none of the loud noises or the voices that are heard nearly all the time in the hospital. The two experiences when Mom had been conscious had reaffirmed my thoughts that people, even when dying, are aware of what is going on around them. All conversations about Mom's condition were held in the hallway at my insistence.

Fortunately, the noisy roommate had left and Mom's new roommate, Rose, was considerate. Learning that Mom was near death, when I told her how blessed her silence was in comparison with the prior roommate, she decided not to turn on her TV, even when I tried to encourage her. So, Mom's bedside was generally fairly quiet. I left the room from time to time to scour the hospital for magazines suiting Rose's interests.

But I wanted Mom home and the hospital bed in the living room where Mom would be aware, even if she lacked true consciousness, that she was home with us, that she was loved, and that she was cared for. Alas, this was not to be.

Looking back, not being with Mom when she died was not the worst thing I've ever done, although I certainly grieved about it for weeks after her death. My deepest regrets center on my certainty that if I'd known on September 14, 2000, what I now know, Mom would undoubtedly still be alive.

———

As America watched, the decision whether Terry Schiavo, who had been in a persistent vegetative state since February 1990, would remain on life support—tube feedings—made its way into living rooms across the country in March 2005. What might have been a private decision between a patient's family and her doctors became a cause célèbre as Schiavo lay dying after her feeding tube was removed for the third and final time. Schiavo's parents and family sought to prevent her husband-guardian from ordering that her feeding tube be removed. Without artificial nutrition and hydration, Schiavo would die within one to two weeks. Florida's highest state court decided not to intervene in the decision to end tube feedings. Legislators in Washington D.C. then hurriedly convened to discuss and decide to hand her case over to the federal courts. Eventually, Schiavo's fate was left in the hands of the U.S. Supreme Court, which ultimately decided not to intervene. She died not long thereafter.

The Issue of Tube Feeding

The decision of whether or not to provide artificial nutrition is more controversial than any other intervention. Physicians' ethics committees have stated it is ethical for physicians to discontinue treatment in appropriate cases.[2] In most states, if your loved one has adequate mental capacity, her refusal of artificial nutrition will be honored even though that refusal will lead to death. If she is unable to participate in the decision, you as her patient advocate or health care agent will be permitted to make nutritional decisions consistent with your loved one's previously written advance directive. This right is not limited to patients who are comatose or terminally ill.

You, your loved one, and her physician should consider not just medical reasons why tube feedings should or should not be instituted but also the social, cultural, religious, or psychological significance of withholding or providing such treatment. Caregivers and their loved ones derive social and psychological benefits from hand-feeding. Another consideration is that once a feeding tube is inserted, the decision to discontinue it may be more difficult for you and your family. Many people choose not to be hospitalized or to receive IV hydration, and in some cases antibiotics, should they be near death. But families often experience tremendous conflict between feeling an obligation to sustain life and wanting "nature to take its course."

There are other considerations. Your loved one's nutritional needs may be better met by a feeding tube, but perhaps hand-feeding provides prolonged interaction between you and her that may better meet her needs as a whole, even though hand-feeding poses risks of aspiration, pneumonia, and death. Hand-feeding may help your loved one adjust to the idea of imminent death and may allow family caregivers to begin active grieving. Caregivers and loved ones alike associate hand-feeding with love, compassion, tenderness, and caring. Caregivers may need reassurance that the decision to withhold artificial nutrition, ensuring starvation, does not mean they do not care. On the other hand, your loved one may want tube feeding in order to survive long enough so that a son or daughter who is far away may get to her bedside.

A more difficult problem may be in communicating the decision to withhold nutrition or hydration at the end of life to other family members, such as siblings. Family members may need assurance that it is not morally wrong. Religious beliefs are often cited as a reason why tube feeding is required; some believe that failure to provide sustenance is immoral.

The Orthodox Jewish religion has decreed that life-sustaining treatment is reasonable only if the patient's quality of life is sufficient to justify prolonging her life. As was made clear recently in the widely publicized Schiavo case, the stance of the Roman Catholic Church appears to be evolving. Whereas previously, the Church appeared to approve withholding tube feeding if it would merely prolong suffering,[3] Pope John Paul II has since said that feeding tubes are "morally obligatory" for most patients in persistent vegetative states. Referring directly to Schiavo during the controversy that arose when her feeding tube was removed for the third and final time in March 2005, high ranking cardinals said that removing her feeding tube could lead to legalized euthanasia.[4]

Family members who aren't designated health agents and who've had limited experience in the caregiving for your loved one may find the decision to withhold artificial hydration and nutrition easier to understand if they know that while it may be helpful and in fact lifesaving in many situations, it doesn't provide comfort care for the dying patient. Experience has shown that there is no pain associated when dying patients are not given artificial hydration or food. In fact, most dying patients stop eating altogether and take in less and less fluid. By giving small sips of water, ice chips, or lubricants for the mouth, caregivers can ease any discomfort or sense of thirst. Patients generally slip into a coma, a sleep-like state that is essentially pain-free.

Tube feedings will, on the other hand, prolong life and may worsen the dying process. Family members should be encouraged to consider their loved one's comfort—both physical and mental comfort—so that a family member's reluctance to follow the written or verbal instructions of the patient is overcome.

Because the decision not to use tube feeding can be a very difficult one to make, a discussion about such life-sustaining measures should take place long in advance of the need to make a decision. You will want to explore whether your loved one's preference for treatment is the same or varies in several different circumstances. If, for example, your loved one suffers a stroke and is unable to speak or walk and her condition will never improve, or if she is diagnosed with incurable cancer that is spreading rapidly, what are her wishes with regard to tube feeding that will prolong her life or her suffering? A lot depends upon her specific condition, her chances of survival, and her quality of life if she survives.

Advance Medical Directives

Some decisions are best not left until the end of life. One of these is the ability to put safeguards in place regarding treatment during last illnesses. If your loved one makes a designation naming you as her patient advocate or health care agent, you will have the authority to direct and empower a physician, nursing home, or hospital to rely upon your treatment decisions if she is unable to participate in those decisions.

These are all good reasons why a written designation should be made, for written designations eliminate the difficulty of end-of-life decision-making. If your loved one is unable to communicate her wishes, serious conflicts may arise when family members are called upon to decide whether tube feeding—or cardio-pulmonary support, or antibiotics, or advanced diagnostics such as a brain biopsy or a spinal tap—should be provided. Indeed, the opinions and biases of some family members may not be consistent with the wishes of your loved one. At other times, emotions such as guilt, grief, or potential conflicts of interest may cloud the issues. If the family doesn't truly understand the issues, they may make decisions that are not only inconsistent with their loved one's condition and probable outcome but that are also contrary to her wishes. This is why it is so important that she make her preferences for care and/or withdrawal of treatment clear.

A proper designation will make tackling decisions for a loved one at the end of life far, far easier and may permit your loved one to die with dignity, for advance directives eliminate any guesswork about what her wishes might have been.

All states have some kind of end-of-life legislation permitting residents to state in advance their wishes for end-of-life care. The document is known by various names such as "Living Will" (although the document is not actually a will), "Durable Power of Attorney for Health Care," and "Advance Directive." In such a document, you loved one will be able to specify the type of care she doesn't want if her physicians say that she's too ill to survive, and she will also be able to tell her doctors how comfortable she wants to be. In other words, she'll be able to specify that she wants enough pain medication to keep her comfortable even if the drugs would hasten her death.

Refusal of Treatment

A patient who has put her wishes about end-of-life care in writing on a proper form may authorize her patient advocate to refuse treatments, even when that will cause the patient to die.

She'll also be able to specify that no cardio-pulmonary resuscitation (CPR) and no extraordinary treatment such as mechanical breathing and artificial nutrition be given to her. She can direct that if such a treatment has already been instituted, it should be withdrawn. If she chooses to have no CPR if her physicians say that her condition is terminal, she might also choose to wear a "DNR" (Do not resuscitate) bracelet. Her chart, when she is hospitalized, will then be marked "DNR."

She will also be able to authorize you to make decisions about if and when such treatments may be used or withdrawn if she puts it in writing in a form that is legally binding in the state where she lives. Fortunately, the laws of most states permit physicians and health care facilities to honor your terminally ill loved one's written directive so long as she was mentally competent when she wrote the directive and as long as her request is not intended to end her life, even if refusing the treatment means that life is not prolonged and death is hastened. "Terminally ill" usually means an incurable or irreversible condition with no possibility of recovery. If she does not have a medical directive, there is no assurance that the physicians or hospital will honor her wishes or permit you to make those decisions if she is unable to do so (if, for example, she is comatose).

In many states, as a family caregiver, you might be permitted to make treatment decisions even if your loved one has not previously expressed her wishes and has not appointed you as her patient advocate or health care agent, but this cannot be guaranteed. States have the right to set their own standards about how decisions can be made for patients who lack the capacity. In some states, certain of these end-of-life decisions may only be made in writing by the patient and no proxy or surrogate decision makers are allowed to make them. For example, the New York State Health Department does not allow a proxy or surrogate to make the decision to refuse or withdraw feeding tubes; only the patient may make this decision. If there is no one to speak for your loved one, a physician can make the decision, within the limits of state law. The physician will also base the decision on what treatment would provide the best outcome for your loved one.

In the case of Jesica Santillan, a 17-year-old girl whose body rejected the heart and lungs transplanted at Duke University Medical Center in February 2003 because the blood type of the donor did not match, physicians removed life support after they determined that she had suffered severe and irreversible brain damage.

In some states, patient's families have been able to demonstrate by clear and convincing evidence a comatose patient's wishes for end-of-life care and treatment and to get treatment withdrawn. In 1986, in a landmark decision by the Supreme Court of Massachusetts, a family was successful in getting their loved one's feeding tube removed when they were able to prove through testimony of disinterested witnesses that he had previously verbally stated his wish not to "live as a vegetable."[5]

But in other cases in other states, families have not been able to demonstrate their loved one's wishes about end-of-life care to the satisfaction of the trial court and their requests to have life support withdrawn have been refused, as in the Missouri case of Nancy Cruzan, who had been in an automobile accident and had remained in a vegetative state for over seven years.

It is thus important and helpful if your loved one's treatment preferences are set forth in an advance directive so that her last wishes may be taken into consideration. Sometimes, as the result of stroke or some other neurologic or medical event, patients may lack not only the capacity but also the voice to communicate their wishes and/or make their own decisions. This may occur even though death is not imminent, as in the case of a severe brain trauma that leaves a patient unable to speak, swallow, or feed herself.

Advance directives must be witnessed, in some states they must be notarized, and in most states the designated agents or advocates must sign a statement accepting the designation and its limits. Your loved one's physician and any other person who provides medical or health care to her may not be a witness. No employee of your physician or of any facility where your loved one is cared for may be a witness. No person who believes she owes him money or who may be her heir may witness the document.

Properly Executed Advance Directives

Advance directives must be witnessed and, in most states, the designated agents or advocates must sign a statement accepting the designation and its limits.

Since not all states have the same laws, it is important to consult with a local attorney to learn the requirements in your own state. Or you can download an advance directive that has been drafted specifically to meet the standards in your state at the website of Partnerships for Caring, Inc. at http://www.partnershipforcaring.org.

Such advance directives may be revoked or changed at any time. It is important that you recognize this fact and that you and your loved one insist upon it. The best way to revoke a designation is to tear it up or destroy it.

One well-known directive is called Five Wishes. Many hospitals distribute this directive, which meets the requirements of the District of Columbia and 35 states. It can be ordered from the Internet at www.agingwithdignity.org/5wishes.html, and there is a list on the website of the states where it is legal. Persons who live in other states should consult with a lawyer in their state to see how the requirements compare. Five Wishes is also available from Aging with Dignity at P.O. Box 1661, Tallahassee, Florida 32302-1661.

Five Wishes contains five sections. Wish One allows your loved one to select a health care agent and an alternate and to authorize her to exercise a given level of decision-making. A detailed list of what she may be authorized to do is included and your loved one may cross out anything she does not want her to do. There is also space to write specific instructions.

Wish Two allows your loved one to tell you and her loved ones just what "life-support treatment" means to her. There is space to write exactly what "extra-ordinary measures" means to her. In addition, she can choose different levels of life support depending on three specific situations: where she is close to death, where she is in a coma and not expected to wake up or recover, and where she is suffering permanent and severe brain damage and is not expected to recover.

Wish Three allows your loved one to tell you and your family how comfortable she wants to be. A long list of options for care and treatment that individuals might naturally want are listed, and she may cross out anything she doesn't want. Thus, the need to anticipate options is already done for her and individualizing the form to her own particular value system is very easy.

Wish Four allows your loved one to tell you and her family how she wants to be treated—whether she wants someone at her bedside, whom she wants there, whether she wants pictures of her family nearby, and so on.

Wish Five is called "What I Want my Loved Ones to Know." This section allows your loved one to give end-of-life messages to you and your family and to address issues related to grieving and funerals or memorial services.

Five Wishes is not only clear, it can be individualized. It is a document that most individuals are comfortable with because it isn't written in "legalese." The Miami Herald called Five Wishes a "living will with a heart and soul."

Having an advance directive and designating a patient advocate or health care agent provides your loved one with assurance that her wishes regarding her last days or hours will be honored. It also helps families make difficult end-of-life decisions about issues that can be distressing to families. Family caregivers may need reassurance that carrying out their loved one's last wishes will not cause her pain and discomfort. This is particularly true if she has expressed a wish that nutrition and/or hydration be withheld or withdrawn.

How to Talk about End-of-Life Care

It's seldom easy to cope with the dying process, but talking about and ultimately putting your loved one's wishes in writing has the potential to make
her final days less traumatic and less stressful for her and for you. Special
significance or poignancy may derive from the moments you spend with
her discussing her choices for care at the end of life.

Certainly, your emotional and financial burdens will be lightened when
your loved one has made decisions about how she wants to spend her final
days. While it would surely be easier to talk about end-of-life care with
your loved one while she is healthy, many caregivers will not have that
option.

How do you approach this issue? Jim Towey, founder of the nonprofit
group Aging with Dignity, which has produced and promoted the Five
Wishes living will, suggests that you begin talking about someone else's
end-of-life care first. But if your loved one is feeling sad about the recent
death of a family member or friend, whether that death was sudden or
occurred after a lengthy illness, it's best to give her time to begin grieving
before launching into a talk about her own wishes. It's best to wait for a
day when your loved one is feeling well. If she has a headache or is feeling
blue, that's not the best time to broach the subject.

Be sure to initiate a discussion when you have time for a meaningful
conversation—at least 30 to 60 minutes. You might decide to have this
discussion together with your loved one's physician, but be sure to check
beforehand to make sure her physician has the time. Many physicians are
now trained in end-of-life care and can be good facilitators. Others who
can facilitate are clergy and mental health professionals.

Find a quiet, private place to have this discussion. Distractions such as
visitors and phone calls are not conducive to this kind of difficult conversation. Usually it's best to have a one-on-one discussion.

If your loved one is diagnosed with a serious illness, she may be ready to
discuss end-of-life care. Even if her illness is not terminal, she may be
encouraged to talk about what kind of care she would want if her condition should worsen.

Before you start a conversation about end-of-life choices, be sure you
have learned about the issues and options such as living wills, advance
directives, and hospice care, but don't come to this discussion armed with
a boilerplate living will or advance directive. Give your loved one time to
think about your conversation and then wait for her to bring up the topic
again. If, after a week or so, she doesn't talk about end-of-life decisions,

you might initiate another discussion. Once you feel she's comfortable with the idea, you can give her an advance directive and go over the choices with her.

Here are some ways you might start a conversation with her about the care she wants at the end of her life:

- I'd like to talk about how you would like to be cared for if you got really sick. Is that okay?
- If you ever got really sick, I would be afraid of not knowing the kind of care you would like. Could we talk about this now? I'd feel better if we did.

Once you've raised the issue, you might ask other questions about specific care:

- Where would you like to spend your final days? If possible, would you prefer to be at home or in a home-like setting?
- Are there any circumstances under which you would refuse resuscitation or life-support measures, such as being in a coma?
- What kind of emotional and spiritual support would you like to have during the dying process?
- If you become too sick to talk with your physicians about your care, who would make decisions?
- Do you want to be kept alive as long as possible, even if that means being in an intensive care unit? If you were terminally ill, would you want medications to relieve pain, even if the drugs might hasten your death?
- How do you want your pain managed? Do you want enough medication to block pain even if it might hasten your death?
- Do you want antibiotics if they will only prolong your death?
- Would you want tube feeding if you were recovering from surgery? If your quality of life were poor and tube feeding would only prolong your life, would you want it? What does "quality of life" mean to you? Under what circumstances would you refuse tube feeding or artificial hydration?
- Have you talked to your physician about your wishes regarding end-of-life care?
- Have you given your physician any written instructions about end-of-life care?

- Do you know what kind of services are provided by hospice organizations?
- What, if any, spiritual support would you like if you become terminally ill?

You should consider not only the medical issues involving use of oxygen, pain medications, antibiotics, mechanical life support, and artificial nutrition but also talk about the kind of care that allows your loved one to have dignity and comfort in her last days. It's also important to talk about memories and forgiveness. You should ask her how she wants to be remembered. Your loved one might have special music in mind or poems she wants to hear at her bedside in her final hours.

Don't forget to be a good listener during this conversation. Don't interrupt her, and be sensitive to her mood. Let her set the pace and support her by affirming her thoughts. Show her you agree by nodding or giving her a comforting touch or hug. Remember that you don't need to have decisions made that day if she is having trouble dealing with the idea of impending death. You may decide to postpone the discussion until another day if she becomes uncomfortable.

You and your loved one may benefit from reading the booklet "Talking About Your Choices," developed with funding from the Robert Wood Johnson Foundation and available at The Partnership for Caring website: www.partnershipforcaring.org/Talking/talking_set.html.

Common Questions Regarding Advance Directives

Common fears individuals express regarding advance directives include the following:

1. *What if I change my mind about the whole thing? Suppose I decide I want to take my chances and do want a respirator after all?*

All advance directives are revocable. You can revoke one by tearing it up or by telling your physician, your nurse, your designated advocate, or your family that you have changed your mind. They are legally bound to respect your revocation.

2. *What if I change my mind about whom I want designated as my advocate?*

All you need to do is to cross out the individual's name and sign and date the page. You can even write in the name of an alternate.

3. What if I change my mind about the kind of treatment I do or do not want?

You can change this as well, in the same manner as changing the advocate.

4. Whom should I designate as my patient advocate?

You will know better than anyone whom you trust to be your patient advocate and to enforce your preferences for end-of-life care. Sometimes family members are too emotionally involved, but people usually designate their children or their spouse. Remember that you cannot name your physician, your nurse, or any health care provider as your patient advocate, and they may not witness the execution of one. You will probably want to designate persons who live close enough to you to actively participate, but that is not necessary as your designation can provide for telephone consultations. In all states, an advocate must be 18 or older (21 in Colorado).

5. Won't my children be angry at having to make a decision to withhold treatment from me if that's what my directive says?

In my experience, most children are relieved that their loved one has taken the decision out of their hands. It may sound like a lot of decision-making, but a good directive is quite explicit about the treatment and diagnostics you do and do not want. Consequently, children generally don't feel guilty as they are only carrying out your wishes, not making decisions on their own. To ensure this, it is important that you provide your child or children with a copy of your directive and take some time to discuss your wishes with them.

6. What other kinds of powers can I give my advocate?

You can empower your advocate to choose physicians or specialists for you; to move you to another state if that is necessary for treatment; to choose a hospital or nursing home for you and to place you there; to authorize or refuse medications, including pain medications; to decide whether medical treatment, including life-sustaining measures and artificial nourishment, should be started, stopped, or not given at all, including artificially provided water, food, or medications; to apply for Medicare or Medicaid benefits for you; and to have access to your medical records and the authority to release them as need be.

7. Will I still need a "Do Not Resuscitate" order if I have a written medical directive?

Some states will require that you have a separate DNR form. Typically these are available from your local office on aging.

8. *Are there any special forms I need to complete to authorize a patient advocate to act on my behalf at any time I am not able to participate in my treatment decisions?*
Yes, each state has its own particular laws regarding medical directives. It is best to consult with a lawyer in your state to make sure you have a form drafted according to state law. Or, as mentioned earlier, download a medical directive and instructions for your state at the Partnership for Caring website at www.partnershipforcaring.org.

9. *What if my family or my physicians refuse to honor my wishes?*
There isn't an easy answer to this question. It's very important that you discuss your wishes with your physician and your family before you need the benefits of a medical directive. If your family doesn't agree with your position and refuses to advocate for your last wishes, you may need to ask a family friend to be your patient advocate. You also might need to change your physician before a conflict arises.

10. *Who should have copies of an advance directive?*
The person or persons your loved one designates as her patient advocate should have a copy, and her physician and a care facility where she may live should also have one. Some hospitals will keep a medical directive on file. It is advisable to see if the hospital your loved one would ordinarily use will do so.

By facing end-of-life issues before the end of life comes, you will help your loved one and yourself, as well as other family members, approach impending death with grace, courage, and in peace.

Epilogue

NOVEMBER 20, 2000

I was with Mom in her hospital room near our home in Traverse City, Michigan. The room was dimly lit, quiet. It had been a day of preparation, for we now knew Mom was dying. I had arranged with the hospice team for delivery of a Zone-aire bed[1] and oxygen to our home; an ambulance would bring Mom in the morning.

I'd spent the day with Bill, Mom's nurse, and Barb, the nurse's aide, preparing Mom for the transfer. I'd helped with her bath. We'd done skin care. Bill had reminded me about counting Mom's respirations every hour and keeping a record of vital signs. He'd reminded me what was normal for respiration and pulse.

Mom didn't have a fever. She was pale. Her body was lying completely relaxed on the bed. This was a distinct change from the rigidity and extreme tremors she'd experienced prior to admission and for the first few days after admission. We'd brought her to Traverse City only 14 days before, having transferred her from the nursing home downstate to a new, local facility after realizing how grave her condition was. She'd only been in the new facility seven days when it became apparent she needed to be hospitalized.

Mom was getting less oxygen today. On Friday she'd been up to 10 ppm, the most she could have without being on a respirator. Now the oxygen was set at 6 ppm.

In the afternoon, I'd sung the songs Mom had always enjoyed hearing from me: "You'll Never Walk Alone" from Carousel and "Somewhere Over the Rainbow" from The Wizard of Oz. This wasn't easy to do. In the 35 years since I'd stopped singing regularly, I'd lost most of my vocal range. I couldn't remember all of the words to "You'll Never Walk Alone." And it was hard to sing because my throat was tight with tears I was trying not to sob out loud.

Last Friday, Kris, Mom's eldest grandchild, had told me that Mom had revealed to him a few years before that she felt guilty about not being a better mother. I was determined to tell Mom about all of the good things she'd done for us—to give her some peace of mind and affirmation.

"Mom, do you remember how we used to go out to Grandpa's and pick currants? I can close my eyes today and see those currant bushes over near the chicken coop. Do you remember how we used to take them into the kitchen and sit on stools at the table, washing and de-stemming them, then making jelly for the next winter? Do you remember those fall days when you taught me how to can tomatoes, peaches, and pears from Grandpa's garden? I used to think it was so interesting that if you dunked the fruit into boiling water, the skins would slip right off. You made what some people think work into fun!

"Do you remember, Mom, how you used to put us kids in the back of the jeep with bushels of apples or boxes of eggs, and we'd go bouncing off to the farmers' market with them on Saturdays?

"Mom, I always love to remember the days we lived in Flushing, during the rationing for World War II. You used to put us three little children into the pram and push it down the hill to the grocers'. He'd collect ration cards from all of his customers and each customer would receive what the family needed the most. Some people preferred cigarettes to sugar. The grocer would make up the grocery orders based on his customers' needs and the customers would come and pick them up.

"When you went to the store, he'd remove the three cushions that covered the storage area in the bottom of the pram and he'd pack it with bags full of milk, sugar, flour, some meat, fruit, veggies, cereals—the things he knew you needed with three small children. I can't imagine how you got the big English pram back up the hill, it must have weighed so much."

A while later, watching Mom lying so still, I felt that I needed to leave. I'd been with Mom all day. I hadn't eaten since breakfast, except for some juice and crackers the nurses had brought me from time to time.

It was now five o'clock. Through the large window, I could see that the sky was already dark. In the lights from the parking lots, I could see snow falling—another slippery 20-mile drive home on twisting, narrow country roads.

I hadn't been to the grocery store for weeks, except quick stops each day after leaving Mom's room to pick up a few items for dinner. I was scheduled to be at home tomorrow at 8:00 a.m. for delivery of the bed and oxygen and training to use both. The supply service had told me the training session would take about an hour.

I thought about leaving, doing enough shopping to last for a week, going home, having dinner, coming back to the hospital, then returning home early in the morning so I'd be there for the training session. I worried about road conditions. A few nights earlier, when I'd been called to the hospital, I'd nearly lost control of the car on a slippery curve. I'd stayed all night at the hospital, both because Mom needed me and because I was afraid to drive home. Yes, I thought, *going home and coming back seems to be what I should do, but the thought of the slippery roads lingered in the back of my mind.*

I was aware that I was not processing information very well. I was having difficulty deciding what to do and when. I wanted to stay; I felt I needed to get some things done before being confined to the house, twenty miles from town, for an uncertain period of time. I felt unsure. Looking back, I realize that I left because I didn't believe Mom was going to die in the hospital. Mom was coming home the next day for hospice care and was going to die in our living room overlooking the woods.

"Mom, your hand is so swollen, so hot." I bent over and gave Mom a light kiss on her cheek. I laid my head next to hers on the pillow and spoke softly into her ear. "Mom, just think about how wonderful it will be to see Kay again." Kay, my older sister, had died of breast cancer 11 years earlier.

"I think Kay's waiting for you at Heaven's gate. And Mom, I need to tell you that Mike died two weeks ago." Mike was my brother-in-law, Betsy's husband. He'd died of lung cancer. We hadn't told Mom because she was so ill and we thought the news would be too upsetting for her. But how could I let Mom be surprised? If there is an afterlife, and she believed there was, she'd be angry if she found out we'd hidden this from her.

"Betsy is doing just fine, Mom. She asked me to tell you she loves you. And Mom, I want to tell you about Michelle (my niece, Jill's daughter and Mom's granddaughter). She's met the nicest man. He treats her so well. She's really, really happy, Mom. And Jill—Mom, she's looking at job opportunities with that firm we talked about before. She's going to be just fine, Mom. You don't need to worry about anyone. Everyone is going to be just fine.

"Mom," I continued, "I think your friend Susie has got the card table set up in heaven and the cards all dealt. I think Daddy and Uncle Bill are just waiting for you to get there to play bridge. I think you and Susie will clean their clocks. "I'm going to go now. I'm going to get some groceries and eat dinner. Then I'll be back to see you. Tomorrow, you'll be coming home with Glen and me. I'll be taking care of you. But right now, I need to get some food."

Glen and I were finally sitting down to dinner at about 9:00 p.m. when the telephone rang. I got up from the table to answer. It was John, my physician, who was also taking care of Mom.

"Jeannie, I called to tell you that your Mom passed away a few minutes ago." "Oh no, oh no!" I leaned against the wall and took a deep breath. Then I spoke into the receiver. "John, I need you to talk to Glen for a minute." I handed the telephone to Glen.

Glen told John what we had just been discussing. "John, the family wants to ask for an autopsy. They're having great difficulty in understanding how their mom could walk into a nursing home with a urinary tract infection and be dead 65 days later. Everyone who's seen Alice—the nurses here, the relatives, and her friends—no one can understand how she could be so fine in mid-September and then go downhill so fast. The family needs some closure on this."

John said, "I think this is an appropriate case in which to ask for an autopsy. We really don't know what the cause of death is. I'll arrange it."

Glen handed the telephone back to me. John asked me if I wanted to go back to the hospital to spend some time with Mom. I told him that I did. "John, could you please do something for me? When Daddy died and we went back to the hospital to see him, his head was laid far back on the pillow with his mouth gaping open. It was such an awful sight. Could you please ask the nurses to close Mom's mouth? It would make such a difference to me." He agreed to do so.

Glen and I left our dinner on the table and got into the four-wheel-drive Explorer. Glen carefully drove over the slippery snow-covered roads and left me at the entrance to the hospital. While he parked, I went immediately to the fourth floor. The elevator doors opened and I turned right and walked down a hallway, then turned right again.

At the nurses' station, I turned down the hallway toward Mom's room. I saw that all of the nurses and all of the aides were standing guard at the doorway to her room. I know that my face was tight with grief. I don't remember saying anything to anybody, but I remember that they made way for me and that I walked through this honor guard into Mom's room. The curtain was drawn around her bed. I removed my parka and went to her side.

It was quiet. No more steady hissing of oxygen. No more beeping of the IV pump. No more ragged breathing. Mom was lying in the center of the bed. Her oxygen mask was gone. Her arms were at her sides, the covers smooth over her. I bent over the side rail. I put my hands on Mom's face, caressed her forehead, her cheeks. Her face was somewhat cooler than I'd expected.

A nurse I did not know came in and said, "Let me lower that side rail for you." She lowered it and left. Mom was lying on the bed, looking perfectly relaxed—as though she were merely asleep. But her mouth was open. Tears rolling down my cheeks, I put my fingers on her upper lip and tried to close her mouth. This did not work because her head was lying level. I took the pillow underneath her head and scrunched it up into a roll. I put this behind the top of her head. With her head tilted more forward, her mouth was not agape.

I took Mom into my arms and pulled her toward me, holding her for a long time. I was astonished at how hot her back was. Compared to her face, her back was burning up with fever. I'm not sure when Glen came in. He stood beside me as I held Mom. I was surprised at the overwhelming emotions Mom's death *evoked in me. I had not expected her death to impact me so profoundly, in such a primal way.*

Finally I stood up, hugged Glen, and thanked him for being there with me. The nurses had arranged Mom's stuffed animals in a row against the bedrail on the far side of the bed. I gathered these into my arms—the little teddy bear and stuffed cat Jill had given her during a previous hospitalization, and a long-legged bunny with floppy ears and a pink sweater with red strawberries on it that I'd bought her in October. I looked around and found the note I'd made for the wall at Mom's head laid out for me on the table. I folded the note and put it into my pocket.

I leaned over, gave Mom my last kiss, and told Glen that it was okay for us to go now. That was the beginning of a period of months during which I awakened in tears every single morning, remembering some of the episodes of terror that Mom had experienced. I wondered how many times she'd had similar experiences when I was not there to comfort her, to assist her in her state of complete helplessness.

It would be many months before I wondered, in a vague sort of way, what the nurses must have thought when they went in to find Mom with her head tilted forward on the pillow that was scrunched up under her.

—⊡—

It has been five years since Mom died. A friend asks me what I've learned in this period. I've learned that geriatric health issues are exceedingly complex. I find myself thinking that the term "vicious circle," while somewhat descriptive, fails to convey the full impact of what the downward spiral can be like when various diseases and conditions are exacerbated by the side effects and adverse reactions caused by the various medications typically combined for treatment in the elderly.

Most important, I've learned how critical it is to observe changes in status so that early intervention occurs if your loved one suffers from any of the common medical complications discussed in this book. I've also learned that family caregivers are often in the best position to notice these changes and to alert their loved one's physicians and nurses of potentially fatal diseases or conditions. Prevention is also a key issue—one that I've tried to emphasize in this book. Think along these lines and you'll do fine—detection, communication, intervention, and prevention.

I cannot stress enough that you are the first line of defense for your loved one, assuming she is unable to participate in health care decisions. Even if your loved one is able to participate, you still will need to take a proactive stance in order to protect her from overmedication, medication error, adverse drug reactions, and the all-too-common problems caused by chronic understaffing in nursing homes: untreated medical conditions, dehydration, and malnutrition. Of course, while you advocate for her care, you will want to be a welcome member of her caregiving team. Enlist the active cooperation of all those who provide care for her. Be involved, be informed, be sensitive, be tactful, be prepared to back up your suggestions, and be open to ideas from all members of the team. Don't diagnose. That is for your loved one's doctor to do. If you try to impose a diagnosis, you might foreclose another possibility. Remember that medical caregivers caregivers have "bad days" too, and be patient if a stressed, over-tired caregiver seems cranky.

I've learned, too, that it is essential to provide as much continuity of care as you can for your loved one. Choosing a nursing home where your loved one's regular physician can practice will help with this continuity. As I stated earlier, your loved one will receive better care from doctors and nurses who are familiar with her. It's simply too difficult for doctors and nurses, in the limited amount of time available, to fully comprehend the implications of changes in status that could signal any one of several potentially deadly complications. A physician familiar with a patient can more readily interpret these changes in status and avert harm. By the time a physician who doesn't know her can get all of the diagnostics done, it could be too late to prevent serious harm to your loved one.

Finally, I've learned that, even in the best of times, we all make mistakes. Don't beat yourself up. Take care of your own needs so that you are at your best when you care for your loved one. There are many community resources available to assist caregivers, as well as a wealth of information available on the Internet. The armies of caregivers need to have courage and confidence. They need to recognize their strengths, acknowledge their weaknesses, find ways to receive respite care, and to make their efforts count.

Quality care of your elderly loved one presents complicated issues, but using the knowledge and tools provided in this book, you can be the best advocate for your loved one. Don't forget that it is the job of doctors and other trained medical personnel to make the ultimate medical decisions for your loved one. While you can make their job easier by providing valuable information gained through your observations, you needn't take responsibility for their decisions. You will do the best you can under the circumstances in which you find yourself.

In the meantime, take advantage of what may be a brief window in time to heal old wounds and to renew expressions of devotion. You needn't expect yourself to be perfect. You only need to do the best you can. No one could ask for more.

I will always be grateful that Mom made her wishes about end-of-life care known to us. She'd also told me that she wanted to be cremated. That had been Daddy's wish as well, and my sisters and I decided that I would scatter Mom's ashes in the same spot as Dad's.

So it was that on a warm, sunny day in December 2000, Kris, Trisha, and their dad, Dan Pahl, met Glen and me at a marina in Florida. We sat on a pontoon boat, telling stories about Nana, remembering her and Papa, and laughing and crying, until we scattered her ashes, following them with a huge heart-shaped wreath covered with pale pink roses and streamers of pink and rose ribbons. When it floated off across the water toward the ocean, it took some, but by no means all, of our pain with it.

—◧—

In spite of illness, in spite even our arch-enemy sorrow, one can remain alive long past the usual date of disintegration if one is unafraid of change, insatiable in intellectual curiosity, interested in big things, and happy in small ways

EDITH WHARTON, *A Backward Glance*

Appendices

Appendix A
Choosing a Nursing Home or Other
Long-Term Care Alternative

Printable pages. Any of the pages in these Appendices may be printed for use on 8.5 x 11-inch paper at www.goodmedicalcare.com.

Administration on Aging: www.aoa.dhhs.gov/
Call (800) 677-1116 to find local services for older Americans.

Your local area agency on aging has free guides and information about such care options as adult foster care homes, adult day care, home health services, assisted living facilities, and long-term care facilities. Additionally, the Medicare/Medicaid options that are available to help your loved one stay in her own home are coordinated through that office.

Find this office in your local telephone directory or call the toll free number above.

U.S. Government Medicare Website: www.medicare.gov
This Medicare website contains a free guide to choosing a nursing home, an interactive site where you can compare nursing homes in your area, a checklist for you to use when touring nursing homes, and information on alternatives to nursing home care.

Medicaid information concerning long-term care services in the United States is found at www.cms.hhs.gov/home/medicaid.asp

Medicare: www.medicare.gov/NHCompare/Home.asp
This is the federal government's official nursing home guide page. It offers pamphlets on how to choose a nursing home and, for the first time, the actual results of nursing home inspections ("surveys") for every Medicare/Medicaid certified nursing home in the country. The "tags" and the names of the problems cited ("deficiencies") and the seriousness ("scope and severity") are posted here. However, the actual text of the citations is not available.

See also www.la4seniors.com/nursing_homes.htm

Appendix A

National Citizens' Coalition for Nursing Home Reform:
www.nccnhr.org/public/50_156_434.CFM
This is the website for the leading citizen's consumer watchdog for long-term care facilities. Many fine articles and fact sheets are available, as well as many links to other websites of interest to long-term care users. News about pending legislation and other topics of interest are prolific.

State Ombudsmen: www.nccnhr.org/static_pages/ombudsmen_list.cfm
You will find all contact information here for your state's nursing home ombudsmen.

Citizen's Groups Supporting Nursing Home Reform:
www.nccnhr.org/static_pages/Citizens_groups_list.cfm
The NCCNHR website has links to citizens' advocacy groups in all 50 states. Many of these groups have on-line information regarding how to choose a nursing home.

Citizens for Better Care of Michigan:
The Citizens for Better Care of Michigan has numerous helpful booklets available on all facets of nursing home care. Many are available free online at www.cbcmi.org/publications.htm

Others may be ordered and the cost is nominal ($2.00 to $3.00). "How to Choose a Nursing Home" ($3.00) is particularly helpful. Go to www.cbcmi.org/publications/nhlook.htm to order this.

A video version is available for $9.00. Go to www.cbcmi.org/publications/video.htm to order this.

Appendix B
Government Programs to Keep the Elderly in the Community

The Health Care Financing Administration (HCFA), charged with oversight of American nursing homes, also oversees government programs that are designed to keep the elderly in their own communities and, if possible, in their own homes.

Some of the assistance provided under these programs includes the Medicaid Home and Community-Based Service Waivers. These waivers allow individual states to develop and implement alternatives to long-term care facility placement. The program is described at www.hcfa.gov/medicaid/hpg4.htm. At the time of this writing, budget cuts are looming and these programs may disappear. Some of the services that currently can be provided at no cost to seniors and disabled persons who qualify include:

1. Case management
2. Homemaker/home health aide services
3. Personal care services
4. Adult day health
5. Rehabilitation
6. Respite care

Other services, if approved by HCFA and requested by the state because they are needed by waiver participants to avoid being placed in a medical facility, include:

1. Non-medical transportation
2. In-home support services
3. Special communication services
4. Minor home modifications
5. Adult day care

For those with chronic mental illness, services (exclusive of coverage for room and board except for certain limited circumstances) include:

1. Day treatment or other partial hospitalization services
2. Psychosocial rehabilitation services
3. Clinic services

You can get more information by telephoning or visiting the agency on aging in your own community or by telephoning your social security office if you need help in finding the right office.

Appendix B

The following websites have valuable information from the U.S. Government Medicare website for Medicaid Waiver & Demonstration Projects.

Medicaid State Waiver Program Demonstration Projects—
General Information
www.cms.hhs.gov/MedicaidStWaivProgDemoPGI/

Medicaid Demonstration Projects & Evaluation Reports
www.cms.hhs.gov/DemonstrProjectsEvalRepts/

Medicaid Health Insurance Flexibility & Accountability (HIFA)
www.cms.hhs.gov/HIFA/

Medicaid Pharmacy Plus
www.cms.hhs.gov/MedicaidPharmacyPlus/

Appendix C
Diagnosing Delerium and Its Underlying Causes

Because delirium can be fatal if the underlying causes are untreated and because an inappropriate diagnosis of dementia may result in failure to treat those underlying causes, it is imperative that delirium and its causes be detected. The following checklist will help you ensure that all diagnostic tests are done. Make sure that you put a copy of this checklist in the three-ring binder in which you are building your loved one's medical history.

STANDARD DIAGNOSTIC TESTS—UNEXPLAINED DELIRIUM

Complete blood count
* Anemia
* Infection

Electrolyte levels
* High or low levels of potassium or sodium
* Dehydration
* Renal (kidney) failure
* Endocrinopathy
* Acidosis

Blood chemistry panel
* Hypercalemia or hypocalcemia
* Hypoglycemia or hypoglycemia
* Liver dysfunction
* Renal (kidney) failure

Urinalysis
* Infection

Electrocardiogram
* Myocardial infarction
* Arrhythmias

Chest X ray
* Pneumonia
* Congestive heart failure

CT Scan
* Cerebrovascular accident

The previous are diagnostic tests for the more common conditions causing delirium. If these tests do not establish a diagnosis, the following tests may be applicable, if justified by the findings of the history and the physical examination and also by the clinical situation:

Blood culture
- Sepsis

Cardiac isoenzyme levels
- Myocardial infarction
- Hypoxia

Arterial blood gases
- Acidosis
- Thyrotoxicosis

Thyroid function tests
- Hypothyroidism

Toxicology screen
- Drug intoxication

Drug levels
- Drug toxicity

Lumbar puncture
- Meningitis

Electroencephalogram
- Seizures

Appendix D
Risk Factors for Delirium

The following are risk factors predisposing the elderly to delirium. Check each of the following factors that applies to your loved one and update this form often. If your loved one has a sudden change in cognition, review this appendix with her nurse and physician to help diagnose delirium.

Medications: The following kinds of medications can cause delirium. How many of them are prescribed for your loved one?

_____ Antipsychotics

_____ Anxiolytics

_____ Antidepressants

_____ Digitalis glycosides

_____ Antiarrhythmics

_____ Calcium channel blockers

_____ Beta blockers

_____ H2 antagonists

_____ Narcotics

_____ Corticosteroids NSAIDs

_____ OTCs with anticholinergic properties

Conditions or Diseases: The following conditions or diseases can predispose your loved one to delirium. Does your loved one have any of these?

_____ **Intoxication** (alcohol or medications)

Infection

_____ Urinary tract infection

_____ Pneumonia

_____ Sepsis

Fluid or electrolyte disturbance

_____ Dehydration

_____ Acid/base disturbance

_____ Derangements of calcium, potassium, sodium, or magnesium

Metabolic derangement

_____ Hypoxia

_____ Hypoglycemia

_____ Hyperglycemia

_____ Hepatic or renal insufficiency

_____ Vitamin deficiencies

_____ Thyroid or parathyroid dysfunction

_____ Hypercortisolism

_____ Hypocortisolism

Cardiopulmonary disease

- Myocardial infarction
- Congestive heart failure
- Cardiac arrhythmias
- Hypertensive encephalopathy
- Severe hypotension
- Pulmonary embolism
- Chronic obstructive pulmonary disease
- Anemia or acute blood loss

Cerebral disease or event

- Stroke or recurrent temporary ischemic event
- Infection: meningitis, encephalitis, abscess, or encephalopathy occurring in acquired immunodeficiency syndrome
- Hematoma: subdural, epidural, or intracerebral
- Inflammatory disease: temporal arteritis or cerebral vasculitis
- Primary or secondary subarachnoid hemorrhage following trauma
- Nonconvulsive generalized status epilepticus

Miscellaneous events

- Fecal impaction
- Urinary retention
- Hypothermia or hyperthermia
- Environmental change, especially hospitalization
- Trauma
- Burns
- Fractures
- Surgery

Appendix E
Physiological Causes for Behavior Problems

Sometimes an elderly patient's problem behavior is caused by non-psychiatric reasons. To avoid the unnecessary use of an antipsychotic or other psychotropic medication that has deleterious effects on the elderly, use the following checklist to determine if there is any cause for the resident's behavior other than psychosis or another psychiatric disorder. Keep a copy of this checklist in your three-ring binder.

Physical Conditions

___ Pain

___ Fracture

___ Recent injury due to fall or trauma (major/minor)

___ Chronic disease (arthritis, peptic ulcer disease, chronic obstructive pulmonary disease)

Bowel/Bladder

___ Toileting

___ Drying

___ Impaction

___ Catheter discomfort/pain

___ Abdominal distention

___ Bladder enlargement

Disease States

___ Diabetes (low glucose, high glucose)

___ Thyroid abnormalities

___ Urinary tract infection

___ Respiratory tract infection

___ Congestive heart failure

___ Peptic ulcer disease

___ Chronic obstructive pulmonary disease/asthma

Prescription Medications

___ Antipsychotics/anticholinergic agents (Examples: Risperdal, over-the-counter allergy medications)

___ Antianxiety medications (Examples: Valium, Ativan)

___ Cardiovascular agents (heart medications example: Digoxin)

___ Antidepressants

___ Digitalis glycosides (heart medication)

___ Xanthines (caffeine)

___ Narcotic and non-narcotic analgesics

___ H2 blockers (heart medication)

___ Recent change in medications

Over-the-Counter Medications

___ Anticholinergic agents

___ Antihistamines

Environmental Factors

___ Change in environment/strange environment

___ Change in roommate

___ Death/absence of a spouse

___ Stress

___ Too much noise/light

Nutrition

___ Hunger

___ Thirst

Eyes, Ears

___ Decreased vision

___ Decreased hearing

Metabolic States

___ Abnormal electrolytes (sodium, potassium)

___ Blood gases (CO_2)

Neurological Deficits

___ Stroke

___ TIA (mini-stroke)

___ Seizure activity

___ Tumor

___ Trauma

Depression

___ Agitation

___ Irritability

___ Isolation (wish to be left alone)

___ Insomnia

___ Rule out causes such as caffeine intake, poor sleep habits

Positioning

___ Cramped

___ Uncomfortable

___ Restraints

Appendix F
Finding a Geriatric Care Manager

One way to avoid long-term care placement is to retain the services of a geriatric care manager. If you do so, your loved one might be able to avoid nursing home placement.

WHAT IS A GERIATRIC CARE MANAGER?

The geriatric care manager (GCM) is a private practitioner in a relatively new area of practice. GCMs contract independently with families to provide medical oversight for elderly community-dwelling seniors. This service is particularly helpful for adult children who live hours away from loved ones. A GCM is a professional who specializes in assisting older people and their families in meeting their in-home health care and long-term care arrangements. GCMs are trained in gerontology, social work, nursing, and/or counseling. Some of the things a geriatric care manager may do include:

- Acting as a contact person for family members who live at a distance and providing information, support, alerts to problems, and reassurance
- Conducting care-planning assessments to identify problems
- Determining eligibility for assistance and need for services
- Screening, arranging, and monitoring in-home health care or other services
- Taking responsibility for financial, legal, or medical issues
- Arranging or offering referrals to geriatric specialists to avoid future problems
- Taking charge in case of emergencies
- Helping an elderly person find a retirement complex, assisted living, adult foster care home, or nursing home
- Assisting an elderly person with moving from her home to a facility
- Advocating for the elderly with physicians, hospitals, caregivers, and governmental agencies
- Providing counseling and support
- Some geriatric care managers also provide therapy (family or individual), money management, and guardianships or conservatorships. GCMs have extensive knowledge about services for the elderly in their community— availability, cost, and quality.

WHAT ARE THE BENEFITS OF HAVING A GERIATRIC CARE MANAGER?

One of the benefits of having a geriatric care manager is the flexibility of services that may be offered. A contract between a family member and a GCM will be tailored to the specific needs of your family. A GCM can be particularly helpful when you're the leader who coordinates care for an elderly loved one who lives far from your home. Other benefits of having a GCM include:

Short-term or ongoing assistance. This is important for caregivers who live far away.

Services that are individualized. GCMs can offer services that are client-centered and tailored to meet the client's specific wants and needs.

Flexible scheduling. Many GCMs are available after hours and on weekends.

Continuity of care management. GCMs can be the point man, making decisions to reduce miscommunications and to minimize time, stress, and cost to clients.

Avoidance of medical emergencies. GCMs can monitor your loved one's medical, physical, and psychological health consistently and can help prevent costly crises and unnecessary hospitalizations.

Reduction of nursing home care. GCMs can help your loved one to avoid inappropriate and costly institutional care and overuse of services.

To find a geriatric care manager in your loved one's geographic locality, use the search engine at the website of the National Association of Professional Geriatric Care Managers at www.caremanager.org or www.findacaremanager.org

Appendix G
Common Drug-Drug Interactions

The medications listed below are commonly prescribed for the elderly; various drug-drug interactions frequently occur. Be sure to discuss these medications with your loved one's physician and ask about her risk for interactions.

DRUG	PURPOSE	INTERACTS WITH	RISK
Celebrex (celecoxib)	NSAID prescribed for arthritis pain	Other NSAIDS such as aspirin or ibuprofen	Increased risk of ulcers
Celebrex	NSAID prescribed for arthritis pain	ACE inhibitors (ex. Vasotec)	May reduce effect of antihypertensive
Lipitor (atorvastatin calcium)	Lowers cholesterol	Drugs prescribed to suppress the immune system	May increase creatinine levels, causing muscle weakness and pain
Norvasc (amlodipine besylate)	Controls high blood pressure and angina	Viagra (prescription erectile dysfunction medication)	May cause decrease in blood pressure, dizziness, fainting
Prilosec Delayed Reaction Capsules (omeprazole)	Used to treat gastroesophageal reflux disease; eases ulcers and heartburn	Prescription drugs containing diazepam, e.g., Valium	Increases amount of diazepam available in blood; can increase drowsiness
Prilosec Delayed Reaction Capsules (omeprazole)	See above	Prescription blood thinners (Coumadin, warfarin)	May cause abnormal bleeding
Synthroid (levothyroxine sodium)	Thyroid replacement for those with deficiencies	Prescription cholesterol drugs containing cholestyramine or colestipol	Reduces amount of thyroid available in blood; must be taken six hours apart
Synthroid	See above	Prescription blood thinners (e.g., Coumadin, warfarin)	May cause abnormal bleeding

Appendix G

DRUG	PURPOSE	INTERACTS WITH	RISK
Synthroid	See above	Tricyclic antidepressants such as Elavil	Enhances effects of both drugs, nervousness
Vicodin (hydrocodone bitartrate and acetaminophen)	Narcotic pain reliever, treats moderate to severe pain	Drugs containing other narcotics and Acetaminophen	May suppress the central nervous system (CNS), causing mental and physical impairment and irregular breathing
Vicodin	Narcotic pain reliever, treats moderate to severe pain	MAO inhibitors (a type of antidepressant)	May increase effects of antidepressant; may suppress CNS
Xanax (alprazodam)	Used to treat panic disorder, anxiety, insomnia	Other psychotropics	May suppress CNS, causing confusion, impaired concentration, and coordination
Xanax	See above	Prescription anticonvulsants	See above
Xanax	See above	Antihistamines	See above
Zoloft (sertraline HCl)	Used to treat depression, panic disorder, obsessive-compulsive disorder, and post-traumatic stress disorder	MAO inhibitors, a type of antidepressant such as Marplan, Nardil, Parnate	May cause an elevation in blood pressure, sudden fever, and even death. Zoloft should not be used within two weeks of starting/ stopping an MAO inhibitor
Zoloft	See above	Prescription blood thinners	May cause abnormal bleeding
Zoloft	See above	Prescription triptan migraine drugs	Stimulates constriction of blood vessels; may raise blood pressure and cause coordination problems

Appendix G

Common over-the-counter (OTC) drugs and herbal remedies such as those listed below also frequently interact with medications commonly prescribed for the elderly. Be sure your loved one tells her physician if she is taking any of these compounds and be sure she asks her doctor about the potential for interactions.

DRUG	PURPOSE	INTERACTS WITH	RISK
Advil (ibuprophen)	NSAID prescribed for fever and for pain and stiffness caused by osteoarthritis and rheumatoid arthritis	Blood pressure medications	May cause edema (fluid retention) and swelling
Advil	See above	Prescription blood thinners	May cause abnormal bleeding
Advil	See above	Prescription or OTC drugs containing aspirin	May increase side effects of Advil such as stomachache
Aleve (naproxen sodium)	Reduces inflammation and pain; reduces fever	Prescription or OTC drugs containing aspirin	Increases risk of intestinal bleeding
Aleve	Reduces inflammation and pain; reduces fever	Prescription blood thinners such as Coumadin, warfarin	May cause abnormal bleeding
Aleve	See above	Herbal supplement ginkgo biloba	May cause severe intestinal bleeding
Bayer Aspirin	To reduce blood clots; to ease pain and inflammation	Prescription blood thinners	May cause abnormal bleeding
Bayer Aspirin	See above	Prescription blood pressure medications	May enhance effect of blood pressure meds
Bayer Aspirin	Reduces blood clotting; eases pain and inflammation	Prescription or OTC meds with ibuprophen or naproxin	Increases irritation of stomach lining

DRUG	PURPOSE	INTERACTS WITH	RISK
Benadryl Allergy & Cold (diphenhydramine HCL and acetaminophen)	To relieve symptoms of allergy; reduces cold symptoms	Prescription or OTC meds containing diphenhydramine or other antihistamines	Increases drowsiness, may cause sedation, dizziness, low blood pressure
Benedryl Allergy & Cold	To relieve symptoms of allergy; reduces cold symptoms	Prescription medications that sedate such as Xanax, Valium	Drowsiness, sedation, dizziness, low blood pressure
Benedryl Allergy & Cold	See above	MAO inhibitors (a type of antidepressant)	Drowsiness, sedation, dizziness, low blood pressure
Benedryl Allergy & Cold	See above	OTC sleeping medications such as Sominex	See above
Imodium A-D (loperamide HCl)	To control diarrhea	Antibiotics (cephalo-sporins, erythromycian, tetracycline)	Suppresses effects of Imodium, prolonging diarrhea
Imodium	To control diarrhea	All prescription narcotic pain relievers	Enhances effect of Imodium; risk of severe constipation
Metamucil (psyllium husk)	Adds fiber to diet; to relieve constipation	All prescriptions containing digoxin (to treat congestive heart failure and arrhythmia)	Interferes with absorption, reducing effectiveness of heart meds
Metamucil	Adds fiber to diet; to relieve constipation	All prescription and OTC drugs containing aspirin	Interferes with absorption, reducing effectiveness of aspirin
Pepcid AC (famotidine)	Relieves and prevents acid indi-gestion, heartburn	All OTC antacids taken within one hour of Pepcid AC	Effectiveness of Pepcid AC is reduced

DRUG	PURPOSE	INTERACTS WITH	RISK
Tums (calcium carbonate)	See above	Prescription drugs containing tetracycline	Interferes with absorption and reduces effectiveness of these Rx drugs.
Tums	Relieves and prevents acid indigestion, heartburn	Prescription hypertension meds	Interferes with absorption and reduces effectiveness of Rx drugs. Take Tums one hour before or two hours after
Tums	See above	OTC drugs containing calcium carbonate (e.g., Citracal, Caltrate)	May lead to serious calcium overload and kidney failure
Tylenol (acetaminophen)	To reduce fever and minor pain	Any prescription or OTC NSAID or other drugs containing acetaminophen	Overuse leads to kidney and liver failure; use four grams daily or less
Tylenol	See above	Rx blood thinners	Abnormal bleeding

Appendix H
Medical History

The following questions are relevant to establishing a baseline for your loved one's health. Complete this chart and use it in your three-ring binder as your own medical record. Update it periodically, at least once a month and preferably once a week, or whenever you observe a change in the physical or mental status of your loved one. Remember, your loved one should be weighed once a week at the same time of day, on the same scale, wearing the same or similar clothing.

Today's Date

Name

Birthdate   **Age**

Height   **Weight**

Body weight   one month ago   six months ago

Has this patient lost five lbs. or 5% in one month?

Has this patient lost 10 lbs. or 10% in the past six months?

Body Mass Index (Trigger: Greater than 27? Less than 22?)

Vital signs (Normal for this individual)

Respiration   **Blood pressure**

Temperature   **Pulse**

Immunization history (Date of last shot)

Tetanus   Pneumococcal vaccine

Influenza vaccine

Recent illness(es); hospitalization(s)   *Attach discharge summary(ies)*
Dates   *Diagnosis/Illness/Hospitalization (reason for)*

Date of last blood transfusion

Anesthesia

Complications of illness/operation(s) in past year

Screening tests in past year [Insert dates]

structural colon studies   lipid levels

electrocardiograms and stress tests

mammograms   Pap smears

prostate examination

prostate-specific antigen levels

ordinary laboratory tests (creatinine, glucose, hemoglobin)

Who has records of these tests? [Attach if possible]

Eating habits: It will be helpful if you keep a checklist recording your loved one's eating habits in the three-ring binder that you are assembling. When you note changes in these habits, you may want to re-evaluate for protein/energy malnutrition.

(Check all that apply)

___ Does not have enough food to eat each day

___ Usually eats alone

___ Does not eat anything on one or more days each month

___ Has poor appetite

___ Is on a special diet

(Eating habits continued)

___ Eats vegetables two or fewer times daily

___ Consumes milk or milk products once or not at all daily

___ Consumes fruit or fruit juice once or not at all daily

___ Eats breads, cereals, pasta, rice, or other grains five or fewer times daily

___ Has difficulty chewing or swallowing

___ Has more than one alcoholic drink per day (if female); more than two drinks per day (if male)

___ Has pain in mouth, teeth, or gums

___ Uses tobacco

___ Drinks coffee/other caffeinated drinks

Chronic diseases or conditions

Name of disease/condition   Date diagnosed   Physician   Medication(s)

_____

_____

_____

_____

Current medications, including prescription and nonprescription drugs, health aids, and over-the-counter products, including vitamin supplements

NAME	DOSAGE	SCHEDULE	DURATION	PRESCRIBER

Appendix H

Are there any medications you have stopped? If so:

NAME	DOSAGE	DATE STOPPED	REASON STOPPED

Does this individual have any known drug allergies? What type of reaction was experienced? For each drug this individual may be allergic to, state the following:

NAME	DOSAGE	DATE OF REACTION	TYPE OF REACTION

Has this individual experienced any of the following in the past year?

___ Sodium and potassium depletion associated with diuretic use

___ Extrapyramidal symptoms resulting from use of psychotropic
    medication(s)

___ Gastrointestinal bleeding caused by aspirin or other NSAIDs

___ Falls associated with medication use

___ Hemorrhagic reactions from heparin and warfarin

Does this individual experience any of the following?

Condition   *How Long?*

___ Gastrointestinal bleeding caused by aspirin or
    other NSAIDs   _____

___ Dependence in activities of daily living
    (esp. eating and dressing)   _____

___ Bladder or bowel incontinence   _____

___ Dementia or delirium   _____

Does this individual experience any of the following?

Condition   *How Long?*

___ Need for home health services   _____

___ New or complex drug regimens   _____

___ Need for rehabilitative services   _____

___ Intravenous therapy or nutritional support   _____

___ Wounds or pressure sores   _____

___ Care of ventilators, stomas, tubes, or appliances   _____

Current symptoms _____

_____

Hearing/vision: Describe any difficulties _____

_____

Mental status

___ Alert

___ Talks logically

___ Awake appropriately

___ Demonstrates logical thinking

___ Memory intact   Short term _____   Long term _____

174

Comments/description: Sleeping habits

___ Alert; sleeps well   hours/night _____

___ Moderate sleep   hours/night _____

___ Sleeps poorly   hours/night _____

___ Sleeps   hours in daytime _____

___ Falls asleep (frequency) _____

___ Falls asleep ___ with ease ___ with difficulty

Comments _____

_____

___ Snores

___ Sleeps in daytime   hours/day _____

___ Uses sleep medication (name of medication) _____

Average day

Patient does these for himself/herself:

___ Gets out of bed

___ Toilets/hygiene

___ Dresses

___ Walks

___ Makes breakfast

___ Eats unassisted

___ Drinks unassisted

Usually or always needs assistance with any of the following:

___ Bathing

___ Dressing

___ Grooming

___ Toileting

___ Eating

___ Walking or moving about

___ Traveling (outside the home)

___ Preparing food

___ Shopping for food or other necessities

Leisure activities / Likes to do the following:

____ Read

____ Watch TV

____ Travel

____ Take walks

____ Socialize

Any emotional difficulties?   Yes _____   No _____

Describe: _____

_____

Any significant stressors

____ Move to different housing

____ Lost spouse

____ Lost job

____ Moved to nursing home

____ Recent stroke

____ Recent surgery

FAMILY MEDICAL HISTORY

Patient's spouse

Name _____ Age _____

Age and date of death _____ Cause of death _____

Patient's parents

Mother's name _____ Age _____

Age and date of death _____ Cause of death _____

Father's name _____ Age _____

Age and date of death _____ Cause of death _____

Sibling's name _____ Age _____

Age and date of death _____ Cause of death _____

Sibling's name _____ Age _____

Age and date of death _____ Cause of death _____

Sibling's name _____ Age _____

Age and date of death _____ Cause of death _____

Sibling's name _____ Age _____

Age and date of death _____ Cause of death _____

Is there any history of dementia in this individual's family?
No _____ Yes _____

If yes, please give details: _____

_____

Symptoms

Does this individual have any symptoms related to the following?
_____ Heart disease
_____ Cancer
_____ Stroke
_____ Infection

Does this individual have any symptoms related to the following?

___ Diabetes mellitus

___ Vision and hearing problems

___ Constipation

___ Sleep difficulties

___ Problems with the feet

___ Incontinence

___ Dizziness

___ Falls

___ Mouth problems

___ Denture problems

___ Swallowing difficulties

___ Arthritis

___ Sexual problems

___ Memory loss

___ Depression

Does this individual experience any of the following?

___ Sadness

___ Crying spells

___ Anxiety

___ Hyperactivity

___ Hostility

Does this individual experience any of the following?

___ Decreased interest in social participation

___ Poor concentration

___ Pessimism about the future

___ Thinking about past

Appendix I
Medication Record

Answer the following questions for every medication your loved one is taking, including over-the-counter medications, "as needed" (PRN) medications, and prescription medications.

Name of the medication

Manufacturer

Date prescribed

Physician prescribing

Condition for which prescribed

Dosage

Schedule

Potential side effects (list or attach package insert)

Optimal dosage for elderly patient

Is this one of the medications having a high risk for adverse drug reactions?
____ Anticonvulsant
____ Antipsychotic
____ Sedative/hypnotic
____ Benzodiazepine-long-acting (half-life > 24 hours)
____ Benzodiazepine-intermediate-acting (half-life 10-24 hours)
____ Narcotic analgesic (Prescription painkiller)
____ Anticholinergic

Manufacturer's precautions

Possible drug-food reactions

Possible drug-drug reactions

Possible drug-disease reactions

Side effects and date first observed

Action taken

Result

Appendix J
Medications and Patient Characteristics That Place Elders at Risk for Adverse Drug Reactions

Below are the specific medications, classes of medications, and patient characteristics that Dr. Mark H. Beers and Dr. Jerry Gurwitz have identified as placing the elderly at high risk for potential adverse drug reactions. You will want to identify each one that applies to your loved one and keep this record in your three-ring binder.

(Check all that apply)

Specific Medications:

___ Digoxin

___ Coumadin, warfarin

___ Lithium

___ Chlopropamide

Class of Medication:

___ Anticonvulsants

___ Antipyschotics

___ Benzodiazepine long-acting (half-life > 24 hours)

___ Benzodiazepine intermediate-acting (half-life 10-24 hours)

___ Narcotic analgesics

___ Anticholinergics

Patient Characteristics:

___ Number of active chronic medical diagnoses (> 6)

___ Number of doses of medication per day (> 12)

___ Nine or more medications

___ Prior adverse drug reaction

___ Low body weight or body mass index (< 22 kg/m2)

___ Advanced age (> 85)

___ Decreased renal function (< 50 ml/min)

Appendix K
Risk Factors Causing Falls

Some factors place a person more at risk for falls than others. Each of the risk factors below is weighted. Put a check in front of each risk factor that your loved one has, then add up the total points. If your loved one scores more than six points, identify him or her as at-risk for falls. You will then need to evaluate ways in which to manage your loved one's risk of falls.

ASSESSMENT OF RISK OF FALLS

Sensory Deficits
____ Impaired speech/language barrier (**1** point)

____ Impaired vision (**2** points)

____ Impaired hearing (**1** point)

Bowel or Bladder Problems
____ Incontinence (**1** point)

____ Diarrhea (**1** point)

____ Frequency (voiding every two hours or less) (**1** point)

Medications
____ Antihypertensive (**2** points)

____ Narcotics (**1** point)

____ Sedatives/Hypnotics (**1** point)

____ Psychotropic medications (**2** points)

____ Antianxiety medications (**1** point)

____ Antiseizure medication (**1** point)

Altered Mental Status
____ Confusion/delirium (**1** point)

____ Hallucinations (**1** point)

____ Seizure within last two months (**5** points)

Previous History of Falls
____ Prior to admission (within one month) (**4** points)

____ Fall during this admission (**6** points)

Impaired Mobility, such as

___ Dizziness (**5** points)

___ Muscular weakness (**5** points)

___ Amputee (**1** point)

___ Paresis (hyperactive reflexes) (**1** point)

___ Uses walker (**1** point)

___ Uses wheelchair (**1** point)

___ Uses crutches (**2** points)

___ Uses cane (**2** points)

TOTAL _____

(More than 6 points? Find ways to reduce her risk for falls.)

Date _____

Time _____

Appendix L
Tools to Monitor Dehydration, Malnutrition, and Kidney Function

In Chapter Seven, you learned about the importance of osmolality as an indicator of dehydration. A valuable part of the medical record you keep for your loved one will be your assessment of his or her hydration status. Using the lab values that you will find in the medical record kept by the nursing home (or by your loved one's physician if your loved one is living independently), you can monitor this status. An important tool is the calculation of osmolality. Keep a copy of this appendix in your three-ring binder and update the osmolality chart frequently.

Calculating Osmolality

	NORMAL	DATE	DATE	DATE
Sodium	135–48			
Potassium	3.5–5.5			
BUN	5–26			
Glucose	65–109			
Osmolality	285–295			

An Internet calculator is found at the following site: www.intmed.mcw.edu/clincalc/osmol.html

You can also calculate this on paper using the following formula:

$$\text{Serum Osmolality} = (2 \times (Na+K)) + (BUN/2.8) + (glucose/18)$$

Because kidney function is adversely affected by dehydration, keeping track of kidney function is important as an early warning that serious problems exist. An important indicator of kidney function is the ratio of BUN to serum creatinine. You can use the lab values in the chart below to make this calculation. Note that a ratio of 20:1 or higher indicates serious kidney malfunction.

Appendix L

Tracking BUN:Serum creatinine ratio

	NORMAL	DATE	DATE	DATE
A. BUN	5–26			
B. Serum creatinine	65–109			
Ratio = (A÷B)/1	< 20:1			

(Normal is < 20:1)

(BUN: Serum creatinine ratio equals BUN ÷ Serum creatinine:1)

Example: 40:2 equals 40 ÷ 2 to 1 (20 to 1 or 20:1)

Another valuable indicator of kidney function measures how well the kidneys filter and eliminate toxins. This is done by measuring the level of serum creatinine left in the bloodstream after filtration. Use the chart below to record lab values and to record the calculation of estimated glomerular filtration.

Calculating Kidney Function—Estimated Glomerular Filtration rate (GFR)

	NORMAL	DATE	DATE	DATE
A. BUN	5–26			
B. Serum creatinine	65–109			
Est. Creatinine Clearance	85–125 (female)			
	95–135 (male)			

A calculator is found on the Internet at www.kidney.org/professionals/kdoqi/qfr_calculator.htm

You can also use the following formula to calculate estimated creatinine clearance:

For men: [[140 - age(yr)]*weight(kg)]/[72*serum Cr(mg/dL)]

For women: [[140 - age(yr)]*weight(kg)]/[72*serum Cr(mg/dL)] X .85

Appendix L

MONITORING BODY MASS INDEX (BMI)

Use the website below to monitor BMI. For this, you will need to keep track of your loved one's weight and height. Again, clinicians recommend that the elderly be weighed once a week at the same time of day, wearing the same or similar clothing.

Body Mass Index

	DATE	DATE	DATE
Weight			
Height			
Body Mass Index (BMI)			

Use the calculator at www.dr-bob.org/tips/bmi.html

Appendix M
Risk Factors for Dysphagia

(Check all that apply)

Age

___ Elderly > 65

Diseases or conditions

___ Gastroesophageal reflux disease

___ Neuromuscular disease, particularly Parkinson's disease

___ Neurologic diseases, such as stroke, depression, and dementia.

___ Hypo- or hyperthyroid diseases, such as Grave's disease

___ Degenerative diseases, such as amyotrophic lateral sclerosis, Multiple sclerosis, Huntington's disease

___ Cerebrovascular accidents

Medication-related side effects

___ Doxycycline

___ Tetracycline

___ Trimethoprim-sulfamethoxazole

___ Long-acting benzodiazepines

___ Phenathiazines (Anti-epileptics)

___ Tricyclic antidepressants

___ Antihistamines

___ Certain antihypertensives (alpha methyldopa, clonidine, and propranolol)

___ Nonsteroidal anti-inflammatory drugs (NSAIDs)

___ Calcium antagonists

___ Nitrates

___ Ascorbic acid

___ Potassium chloride tablets

Appendix N
Monitoring Nutritional Status
and Managing Protein/Energy Malnutrition

Use this checklist to help you monitor for protein/energy malnutrition.
(Check all that apply)

Indicator	Action to take
___ Resident has 5% involuntary weight loss in 30 days, or	
___ Resident has 10% involuntary weight loss in 180 days or less, or BMI is ?21 or less (703 x weight in lbs/height in inches), or	Monitor weight weekly; encourage increased intake
___ Resident leaves 25% or more food on tray in last seven days	

In addition to action taken above

___ Serum albumin <3.4g/dL	
___ Cholesterol<160 mg/dL	Evaluate laboratory tests
___ Hgb<12 g/dL	
___ Serum transferrin<180	

Conditions resident has

___ Takes medications other than multivitamins/minerals	Consult with pharmacist
___ Takes more than three (3) medications daily	
___ Experiences symptoms of depression/anxiety	Ask for assessment
___ Experienced infection (UTI, URI, pneumonia, GI) in last seven days	Begin laboratory tests (urinalysis for infection); review lab work from last 30 days
___ Experienced fecal impaction in last seven days	Implement bowel program
___ Undergoing tube feeding	Contact dietitian for assessment
___ Experiencing functional ADL decline	Consider occupational or physical therapy assessment

Indicator	Action to take
Experiencing difficulty swallowing	Contact speech therapist for assessment and dietician for review of diet for consistency, texture
Developed pressure ulcer in low-risk patient	Begin skin care program
Presence of fever (2° above baseline)	Report to director of nursing, physician
Presence of diarrhea	
Presence of constipation	
Presence of vomiting, nausea	
Presence of dentition problem (ill-fitting dentures, missing teeth, bleeding gums)	Consult dentist

Appendix O
Important Websites

U.S. GOVERNMENT AGENCIES

Administration on Aging
330 Independence Avenue SW
Washington D.C. 20201
(202) 619-7501
www.aoa.dhhs.gov

This federal agency sponsors the Eldercare Locator, an Internet website that identifies area agencies on aging by geographical location. This website is at
www.eldercare.gov or you may call (800) 677-1116 Mon. through Fri., from 9:00
a.m. to 8:00 p.m.

Medicare
www.medicare.gov

Nursing Home Information (Medicare)
www.medicare.gov/nursing/home.asp

Find and evaluate nursing homes in your loved one's community on this website,
or call (800) 633-4227. The Medicare website has information about Medicare eligibility requirements and benefits. A list of participating physicians and information about dialysis facilities, nursing home, and prescription assistance programs is
also found here.

Medicaid
cms.hhs.gov/Medicaid/consumer.asp

Check for eligibility and benefits on this website.

Medicare and Medicaid Program Manuals
cms.hhs.gov/Medicaid
cms.hhs.gov/Medicaid/consumer.asp

ADDITIONAL INFORMATION FOR CAREGIVERS

Assisted Living Federation of America
11200 Waples Mill Road, Suite 150
Fairfax, VA 22030
(703) 691-8100
www.alfa.org

Assistance with geographical locations and listings of accredited housing and
assisted living facilities for the elderly.

Department of Veteran's Affairs
810 Vermont Street, NW
Washington, D.C. 20420
(877) 222-VETS
www.va.gov

Check with the VA to determine whether veteran's health benefits are available for your loved one. Often medications and medical services are available to elderly veterans at low cost or no cost.

Family Caregiver Alliance
690 Market Street, Suite 200
San Francisco, CA 94104
(415) 434-3388
www.caregiver.org

This association provides support and other resources for caregivers.

Hospice Foundation of America
2001 S Street NW, Suite 300
Washington, D.C. 20009
(800) 854-3402
www.hospicefoundation.org

The hospice philosophy and practice is available from this organization.

Hospicelink
1-800-331-1620

This resource provides general information on hospice care and referrals to hospices across the country.

National Hospice and Palliative Care Organization
1700 Diagonal Road, Suite 625
Alexandria, VA 22314
703-837-1500
www.nhpco.org

This organization offers information, patient advocacy, professional education, and referrals to hospice programs throughout the country

National Association of Professional Geriatric Care Managers
1604 North Country Club Drive
Tucson, AZ 85716
(520) 881-8008
wwwcare manager.org or www.findacaremanager.org

Find a professional geriatric care manager through this organization's website.

National Adult Day Services Association
409 Third Street NW
Washington, D.C. 20024
(866) 890-7357
www.nadsa.org

Locate adult day care facilities in your loved one's community at this website.

Eldercare Locator
www.n4a.org

Partnership for Caring
1620 Eye Street NW, Suite 202
Washington, D.C. 20006
(800) 989-9455
www.partnershipforcaring.org

Free state-specific sample forms for durable powers of attorney and living wills are provided by this non-profit organization.

ORGANIZATIONS

Meals on Wheels Association of America
1414 Prince Street, Suite 302
Alexandria, Virginia 22314
(703) 548-5558
www.mowaa.org

You will find meal delivery programs in your loved one's community at Meals on Wheels.

Shepherd's Centers of America
One West Armour Blvd., Suite 201
Kansas City, MO 64111
(800) 547-7073; (816) 960-2022
www.shepherdcenters.org

The Shepherd's Centers train senior citizens to provide part-time respite care. At this time, more than 100 centers are operating around the US.

Visiting Nurse Associations of America
11 Beacon Street, Suite 910
Boston, MA 02108
(800) 426-2547; (888) 866-8773; (617) 523-4042
www.vnaa.org

Obtain information and referrals for home health care and hospice programs at this website.

CONSUMER ADVOCATE GROUPS

National Citizen's Coalition for Nursing Home Reform
1424 16th Street, NW Suite 202
Washington, D.C. 20036
(202) 332-2275
www.nccnhr.org

An organization devoted to promoting quality care in nursing homes, advocating for a resolution to understaffing issues.

State Ombudsmen
www.nccnhr.org/static_pages/ombudsmen_list.cfm

Use this website to locate a state ombudsman, an advocate for residents of nursing homes, board and care homes, and assisted living facilities.

Citizen's Groups Supporting Nursing Home Reform
www.nccnhr.org/static_pages/Citizens_groups_list.cfm

CALCULATORS ON THE INTERNET

The calculators discussed in this book are:
Osmolality calculator: www.intmed.mcw.edu/clincalc/osmol.html
Estimated Creatinine Clearance calculator: www.kidney.org/professionals/
    kdoqi/gfr_calculator.cfm
Body Mass Index (BMI) calculator: www.dr-bob.org/tips/bmi.html

MEDICAL DICTIONARIES

www.medicinenet.com
www.medterms.com/script/main/np.asp

FAMILY MEDICINE JOURNALS

Find the *American Family Physician* (Journal of the American Academy of
FamilyPhysicians) at www.aafp.org/afp/index.html.
Find health information from the American Academy of Family
Physicians at www.familydoctor.org.

The Merck Manuals
www.merck.com/pubs/mmanual
www.merck.com/pubs/mm_geriatrics

ORGANIZATIONS PROVIDING INFORMATION ON SPECIFIC DISEASES AND CONDITIONS COMMONLY AFFECTING THE ELDERLY

ALS Association
2101 Ventura Boulevard
Suite 321 Woodland, CA 91364
(800) 782-4747

Provides information and educational
materials about ALS (Lou Gehrig's
Disease)

Alzheimer's Association
919 North Michigan Ave. Ste. 1100
Chicago, IL 60611
(800) 335-8700
www.alz.org

**American Academy of Hospice and
Palliative Medicine**
11250 Roger Bacon Drive
Suite 8, Reston, VA 20190-5202
(703) 787-7718
www.aahpm.org

American Academy of Opthamology
P.O. Box 7427
San Francisco, CA 94120
(415) 561-8500
www.aao.org

American Diabetes Association
1701 N. Beauregard Street
Alexandria, VA 22311
(800) 342-2383
www.diabetes.org

**American Foundation for
Urologic Disease**
1120 North Charles Street
Baltimore, MD 21201
(410) 727-4400
www.afud.org

American Heart Association
7272 Greenville Avenue
Dallas TX 75231
(800) AHA-USA1
www.americanheart.org

American Lung Association
1740 Broadway
New York, NY 10019
(800) LUNG-USA; (212) 315-8700
www.lungusa.org

American Medical Association
515 North State Street
Chicago, IL 60610
(312) 464-5000
www.ama-assn.org

American Pain Society
5700 Old Orchard Road
First Floor, Skokie, IL 60077
(847) 375-4715
Ass'n of pain physicians.
Referrals to pain clinics, physicians,
support groups

American Parkinson's Disease Ass'n
1250 Blvd., Suite 4B
Staten Island, NY 10305
(800) 223-2732, (718) 981-8001
www.apdaparkinson.com

American Stroke Association
7272 Greenville Avenue
Dallas, TX 75231
(888) 4-STROKE; (888) 478-7653
www.strokeassociation.org

Arthritis Foundation
1330 West Peachtree Street
Atlanta, GA 30309
(800) 283-7800, (404) 872-7100
www.arthritis.org

Cancer Care, Inc.
1180 Avenue of the Americas
New York, NY 10036
1-800-813-HOPE (4673)
In New York, 212-302-2400
www.cancercare.org

Support and education for cancer
patients and caregivers

Cancer Information Service
1-800-4-CANCER (422-6237)

Has 19 offices across the country.
Provides information about cancer
and referrals to hospice, home care,
and support groups

National Cancer Institute
Public Inquiries Office
Chicago, IL 60610
Building 31, Room 10A31
31 Center Drive, MSC 2580
Bethesda, MD 20892
(800) CANCER
www.nci.nih.gov

**National Institute of Neurological
Disorders and Stroke**
Office of Communications/Public
Liason
P.O. Box 5810
Bethesda, MD 20824
(800) 352-9424
www.ninds.nih/gov

National Kidney Foundation
30 East 33rd Street, Ste. 1100
New York, NY 10016
(800) 622-9010
www.kidney.org

National Osteoporosis Foundation
1232 22nd Street, NW
Washington, D.C. 20037-1292
(202) 223-2226
www.nof.org

Parkinson's Disease Foundation
1359 Broadway, Ste 1509
New York, NY 10018
(800) 457-6676 (212) 923-4700
www.pdf.org

Appendix P
Recommended Readings

The following articles are recommended for reading as the topics are universally relevant to those with loved ones in long-term care. You may access these articles in one of several ways. The simplest method would be to use the Internet, typing in the Universal Reference Locator (URL) given for each article. If you have no access to the Internet, take this list to your local library and ask the librarian at the reference desk to provide you with the articles. Typically, the library will provide these at a nominal cost, usually $.10 to $0.25 per page. Finally, you can use the addresses provided below to order reprints from the publishers.

Some of the articles must be read with Adobe Acrobat Reader, which you may download to your computer at www.adobe.com/products/acrobat/readstep2.html

The following articles are recommended for reading as the topics are universally relevant to those with loved ones in long-term care. You may access these articles in one of several ways. The simplest method would be to use the Internet, typing in the Universal Reference Locator (URL) given for each article. If you have no access to the Internet, take this list to your local library and ask the librarian at the reference desk to provide you with the articles. Typically, the library will provide these at a nominal cost, usually $.10 to $0.25 per page. Finally, you can use the addresses provided below to order reprints from the publishers.

1. **Burger, SJ, Kayser-Jones J, Prince J. "Malnutrition and Dehydration in Nursing Homes: Key Issues in Prevention and Treatment."** *Commonwealth Fund.* 2000 July; Pub No 386.
    The authors of this article state that malnutrition, dehydration, and weight loss in nursing homes constitute one of the largest, silent epidemics in this country. According to studies using a variety of measurements and performed over the last five to 10 years on different nursing home subgroups have shown that from *35 percent to 85 percent* of U.S. nursing home residents are malnourished. *Thirty to 50 percent* are substandard in body weight. In fact, according to the authors, the level of malnutrition and dehydration in some American nursing homes is similar to that found in many poverty-stricken developing countries where inadequate food intake is compounded by repeated infections. The consequences of these conditions for elderly nursing home residents are potentially serious.

    The authors hypothesize that most cases of malnutrition and dehydration can be prevented or reversed, if they occur, with the use of an interdisciplinary approach. Physicians, nurses, speech pathologists, dietitians, dentists, administrative nursing home personnel, and CNAs must collaborate in resolving these problems.

    Higher staff-to-resident ratios, both at mealtime and 24 hours a day, are imperative. CNAs must be taught how to assist residents with eating, and knowledgeable registered nurses must supervise them during mealtimes. Not only may malnutrition and dehydration result in readmission to the acute hospital—a stressful event for frail elders—but they also contribute to a decreased quality of life, morbidity, and mortality. In addition to these physiological, psychological, and pathological consequences, nursing home residents who do not receive adequate nutritionand hydration during the last months or years of their lives are denied one of life's greatest pleasures—the enjoyment of food and drink of their choice in a pleasant, social environment. www.nccnhr.org/pdf/burger_mal_386.pdf

Order a free copy of this 50-page report by telephoning the Commonwealth Fund, Communications Department, at 212/606-3800 or writing the Commonwealth Fund, 1 East 75th Street, New York, New York 10021 (Specify Publication No 386).

2. Weight Loss in the Nursing Home Clinical Practice Guideline.

This valuable resource is based upon the Council for Nutrition: Nutrition Literature Resource Compendium in Supplement to Annals of Long-Term Care, 2001; the Merck Manual of Geriatrics, Nutrition, 2nd Edition, 1995-1999; and also the research and work of various doctors including Dr. John E. Morley; Dr. D.R. Thomas; Dr. H. Kamel. www.ltcpractice.com/content/node-6/clinicians/weight.htm

3. Kamel HK, Thomas DR, Morley JE. Nutritional deficiencies in long-term care: Part II management of protein energy malnutrition and dehydration. *Annals of Long-Term Care.* 1998 July;6(7):250.

4. The Silent Epidemic. *American Society of Consultant Pharmacists.* 1998 Aug.

From the American Society of Consultant Pharmacists, The Silent Epidemic identifies specific types of medication-related problems frequently experienced by the elderly. This is a valuable resource for caregivers.

From the Foreword:

When medications are prescribed for patients, the intent is to improve the patient's quality of life by curing a disease, reducing or eliminating the symptoms of a disease, arresting or slowing a disease process, or preventing a disease or its symptoms from appearing in the first place (Hepler and Strand, 1990).

But a medication is a two-edged sword; it can cut both ways. The same dose of a medication given to two different people may cure one and harm the other. In recent years there has been a growing recognition in clinical literature, in the popular press, and in health policy circles that misuse of medications is creating serious health problems, disabilities, and death at an alarming rate. This "silent epidemic" can appear in a variety of situations—when a person is prescribed the wrong medication for his or her medical condition or age, the right medication in the wrong dose, or two or more medications that interact with dangerous, unintended side effects. Eight general categories of medication-related problems have been identified. The resulting physical and mental effects can make people feel worse instead of better, less functional, more confused, and less able to care for themselves. Medication-related problems occur most often in older people and are generally more severe. www.ascp.com/medhelp/silentepic.shtml

5. **Alliance for Aging Research.** *Medical Never-Never Land: 10 Reasons Why America is not Ready for the Coming Age Boom.* 2002.
   From the Foreword:

   This is the Alliance's third report to the nation on the   shortage of health professionals trained to care for the nation's older patients. This study, however, is different from the earlier reports in three fundamental ways.

   - This report focuses on the health professions team, not on physicians or geriatricians only. Appropriate care of the elderly requires a team of health professionals. The shortages we document are equally severe in nursing, pharmacy, social work, and indeed all the allied health professions.
   - By no means do we say that every elderly individual should receive care from a geriatric specialist. We do, however, suggest that every health care provider who treats elderly patients requires some specialized training.
   - Time is running out. Baby Boomers, who begin to turn 65 in a decade, will make a serious problem today practically impossible to solve in a few years. This report identifies 10 reasons why our nation has not yet addressed this critical issue. Behind these barriers are three inconvertible facts:
   - The numbers of older Americans have never been greater, and are about to soar.
   - The numbers of health professionals with some formal training in caring for the elderly are woefully inadequate even for today's population.
   - The American people expect this problem to be fixed for themselves and their families. A recent survey conducted for the Alliance by Opinion Research Corporation shows that three out of every four Americans feel it is very important that their healthcare providers have some specific training to care for the elderly.

   www.agingresearch.org/advocacy/geriatrics/02016_aar_geriatrics_text.pdf

6. *The State of Aging and Health in America*. Merck Institute of Aging and Health and the Gerontological Society of America. 2002.
   The State of Aging and Health report consists of five sections:
   The first section of the report, *The Health of Older Americans*, presents data that illustrate changes that have taken place during the past two decades in several important measures of older Americans' health. Five key measures show trends in life expectancy, death rates, chronic disease, disability, and self-related health status.

The second and third sections present the national and state-by-state *Report Card on Healthy Aging*. The Report Card includes 10 indicators divided into three groups:

- Health Behaviors
- Preventative Care and Cancer Screening
- Fall-Related Deaths and Injuries

The *Report Card* grades the nation and the states based on targets set for the older population in Healthy People 2000, a national effort to improve health by establishing health targets and measuring progress. The Report Card uses a "Pass" or "Fail" grading system based on whether the nation and states met, or failed to meet, a target.

The fourth section or the report, Mental Health and Aging, presents challenges in treating mental illness among the elderly. The section focuses on the treatment of depression in later life, because most research on mental health services and the management of mental disorders relates to depressive disorders.

The fifth section, Training the Health Care Workforce—Present and Future, focuses on the growing gap between older Americans' health care needs and the knowledge of health professionals who care for them. www.agingsociety.org/agingsociety/pdf/state_of_aging_report.pdf

7. Liberalization of the Diet Prescription Improves Quality of Life for Older Adults in Long-Term Care, Vol. 105, Issue 12, Pages 1955-1965 (December 2005. From American Dietetic Association

This article, from the American Dietetic Association (ADA), states the association's position that the quality of life and nutritional status of older residents in long-term care facilities may be enhanced by liberalization of the diet prescription. The Association advocates the use of qualified dietetics professionals to assess and evaluate the need for medical nutrition therapy according to each person's individual medical condition, needs, desires, and rights.

Nutrition care in long-term settings must meet two goals: maintenance of health and promotion of quality of life. This article explores the need for assessment of nutritional status through development of an individualized nutrition intervention plan. The Association stresses the need to balance medical needs and individual desires and maintain quality of life. The Association also stresses the need to consider that food is an essential component of quality of life. Balancing risks vs benefits of therapeutic diets is important. If the food is bland, unacceptable, or unpalatable, this can create risks for poor food and/or fluid intake, resulting in risk of weight loss and undernutrition and a spiral of negative health effects. Allowing the elderly to participate in diet-related decisions can increase their quality of life, and reduce the risks of weight loss and undernutrition and a spiral of negative health effects. www.eatright.org/cps/rde/xchg/ada/hs.xsl/advocacy_adar 0902_ENU_HTML.htm

Appendix Q
Prescribing Psychotropic Medications for Nursing Home Residents

When physicians in a nursing home prescribe a medication for a resident, they intend to improve the resident's quality of life by curing a disease, eliminating or minimizing the symptoms of a disease, slowing or halting the progress of a disease, or preventing a resident from developing a disease or symptoms of a disease. Therefore, federal law (OBRA) requires that physicians apply a benefit-risk analysis in each decision to prescribe a medication. The doctor must decide whether the medication will benefit the *particular resident* enough to warrant the risks the medication may pose to the *particular resident*.[1] Thus, dosages must be tailored carefully to allow for particular patient characteristics taking into consideration the possibility that the drug may interact with that patient's other medications or disease processes.

Because psychotropic medications pose such a threat to the safety of the elderly, federal law strictly regulates the use of psychotropic medications in nursing homes. In order to assist facilities in their compliance with the law, guidelines have been established for the use of psychotropic medications. All of these medications are subject to the "unnecessary drug" restrictions of OBRA. Under these restrictions, medications that are duplicative, excessive in dose or duration, or used in the presence of adverse effects or without adequate monitoring or indication are defined as "unnecessary drugs" that may not be used.[2]

INAPPROPRIATE USES OF PSYCHOTROPIC DRUGS

Under these legally binding OBRA guidelines, the following are inappropriate reasons for use of psychotropic drugs in nursing homes:

- Wandering
- Poor self-care
- Restlessness
- Impaired memory
- Anxiety
- Depression

1. Omnibus Budget Reconciliation Act of 1987: subtitle C, nursing home reform: PL100–203. Washington, D.C.: National Coalition for Nursing Home Reform, 1987.
2. One review found that specific guidelines requiring appropriate diagnosis, target symptom documentation, and reasonable dosage level were widely followed, with compliance rates ranging from 70 to 90%. However, sadly, less specific guidelines that require attempts to use nonpharmacologic interventions and the monitoring of drug efficacy and safety were not widely followed, with compliance rates below 55%. Kidder, SW, supra.

- Insomnia
- Unsociability
- Indifference to surroundings
- Fidgeting
- Nervousness
- Uncooperativeness
- Unspecified agitation or agitated behaviors that do not pose a threat to the resident or to others[3]

APPROPRIATE USES OF PSYCHOTROPIC DRUGS

The following are appropriate reasons for use of psychotropic medications:

- Schizophrenia
- Schizoaffective disorder or delusional disorder
- Psychotic mood disorder
- Acute psychotic episodes
- Brief reactive psychosis
- Atypical psychosis
- Tourette's syndrome
- Huntington's disease
- Organic mental syndromes, including dementia, that have associated psychotic and/or agitated features[4] including specific behaviors such as kicking, biting, or scratching that are quantitatively documented by the facility, cause the resident to present a danger to self or others, or actually interfere with the facility's ability to provide care; as well as continuous crying out, screaming, yelling, or pacing if those behaviors cause an impairment in functional capacity and are quantitatively documented

FEDERAL REGULATIONS FOR PRESCRIBING PSYCHOTROPIC MEDICATIONS

To comply with federal law when prescribing a psychotropic drug, a nursing home must do all of the following:

1. Quantitatively and objectively document the behaviors showing:

- all methods that the facility has tried in order to protect the resident from harming either herself or a third party without using drugs

3. Kidder SW. Regulation of inappropriate psychopharmacologic medication use in U.S. nursing homes from 1954-1997: Part I. *Annals of Long Term Care Online.* Vol 1. 1999 Jan. www.mmhc.com/nhm/articles/NHM9901/kidder.html

4. Gurvich T, Cunningham JA. Appropriate use of psychotropic drugs in nursing homes. *Am Fam Physician.* 2000 Mar 1;61(5):1437-46. www.aafp.org/afp/20000301/1437.html

- that the facility has observed the resident and concluded that the behavioral symptom requires some form of intervention
- that the staff has investigated to determine whether the behavior is caused by other events in the resident's life (e.g., a death in the family)

2. **Demonstrate that the behaviors are persistent or permanent rather than transitory.**

3. **Demonstrate that the behaviors are not caused by preventable reasons such as:**

- Environmental factors (i.e., excessive heat, noise, and overcrowding)
- A change in the resident's customary daily routine
- A change in the resident's medical condition such as constipation, fever, infection, or medication reactions
- Present a danger to herself or to others
- Continuously scream, yell, or pace if these specific behaviors cause an impairment in functional capacity
- Experience psychotic symptoms (hallucinations, paranoia, delusions) not exhibited as dangerous behaviors or as screaming, yelling, or pacing but that cause the resident distress or impairment in functional capacity[5]

4. **Document diagnoses and specific target symptoms or behaviors identified by a physician.** This is because treatment with psychotropic medications is indicated only to maintain or improve functional status.

5. **Monitor the effectiveness of drug therapy.**

6. **Observe dosage limits, typically half of a normal adult dosage or less.** Because the elderly have reduced kidney function and since most psychotropic medications are excreted through the kidneys, this means the elderly are most at risk if given psychotropics.

- Attempt periodic dosage reductions or drug discontinuations
- Monitor side effects, particularly those of antipsychotics

5. Federal regulation, 42 CFR § 483.25(l)(2)(i), Medicare and Medicaid Requirements for Long-Term Care Facilities.

Glossary

Note: If you don't find the word or phrase defined here, use one of the following online medical dictionaries: http://cancerweb.ncl.ac.uk/cgi-bin/omd?action=Home&query= or http://www.medicinenet.com/Script/Main/AlphaIdx.asp?p=A_DICT.

Acidosis. Too much acid in the blood and body, a distinctly abnormal condition caused by the accumulation of acid or the depletion of alkaline reserves. Acidosis is associated with serious diseases or conditions such as diabetic ketoacidosis and severe kidney disease.

Activities of daily living (ADL). The things we normally do in daily living including any daily activity we perform for self-care (such as brushing our teeth, feeding ourselves, bathing, dressing, grooming), work, household tasks, and walking and other leisure activities. The ability or inability to perform ADLs can be used as a very practical measure of ability/disability in many disorders.

Adverse drug reaction. An adverse drug event or drug interaction that results in an undesirable or unexpected event that requires some change in the clinician's care of the patient, such as discontinuing a drug, modifying a dosage, prolonging hospitalization, or administering supportive treatment. ADRs do not include drug withdrawal, drug-abuse syndromes, accidental poisonings, or complications of drug overdose.

Akathisia. A frequent and common adverse effect of treatment with antipsychotic (neuroleptic) drugs. This syndrome consists of subjective (feelings of inner restlessness and the urge to move) as well as objective (rocking while standing or sitting, lifting feet as if marching on the spot, and crossing and uncrossing the legs while sitting) components.

Akinesia. Impaired or non-existent body movement; without movement (or without much movement). In neurology, the term is used to denote the absence (or poverty) of movement.

The word "akinetic" comes from the prefix "a" meaning "without" plus the Greek word "kinesis" meaning motion. A person in a coma is "akinetic."

Amyotrophic lateral sclerosis. Also called ALS or Lou Gehrig's disease. Amyotrophic lateral sclerosis is a classic motor neuron disease. These diseases are progressive chronic diseases of the nerves that come from the spinal cord responsible for supplying electrical stimulation to the muscles. This stimulation is necessary for the movement of body parts. ALS is progressive and fatal. Death usually is not directly related to ALS, but results from simultaneous additional illnesses that ultimately occur because of weakness of the body. These illnesses are often infections.

Anabolism. A constructive, energy-consuming metabolic process; the process of cellular construction and synthesis of protein.

Angina. The chest discomfort that occurs when there is insufficient blood oxygen supply to an area of the heart muscle. Usually, the lack of blood supply is due to a narrowing of the coronary arteries as a result of arteriosclerosis. Common symptoms are a squeezing, pressure, heaviness, tightening, or aching across the chest, particularly behind the breastbone. Pain often radiates to the neck, jaw, arms, back, or even the teeth.

Anorexia. Loss of appetite, a side effect of many medications, particularly psychoactive medications.

Anticholinergic. To block the transmission of acetylcholine. Anticholinergic drugs affect the proper functioning of the cholinergic system, which involves neurotransmitters in the brain similar to those transmitting serotonin or dopamine. However, the neurotransmitters in the cholinergic system transmit acetylcholine. As with the other neurotransmitters, a balance is required for proper functioning. Because these drugs represent a significant risk factor for adverse drug reactions, because elderly persons with multiple concurrent diseases or medical conditions usually take numerous medications to treat these concomitant diseases, and because it is not uncommon for several of these medications to have anticholinergic effects, it is necessary to carefully monitor the patient to avoid drug toxicity. The most common side effects of anticholinergic medications are constipation, urinary retention, blurred vision, dry mouth, confusion, sedation, and orthostatic hypotension.

Anxiolytic. A medication prescribed to lessen anxiety, such as Valium, Xanax, Ativan, etc.

Arrhythmia. An abnormal heart rhythm. The heartbeats may be too slow, too rapid, too irregular, or too early. Rapid arrhythmias (greater than 100 beats per minute) are called tachycardias. Slow arrhythmias (slower than 60 beats per minute) are called bradycardias. Irregular heart rhythms are called fibrillations (as in atrial fibrillation and ventricular fibrillation).

Autonomic nervous system. Part of the nervous system that was once thought to be functionally independent of the brain. The autonomic nervous system regulates key functions of the body including the activity of the heart muscle (see below), the smooth muscles (e.g., the muscles of the intestinal tract), and the glands.

The autonomic nervous system has two divisions: (1) the sympathetic nervous system that accelerates the heart rate, constricts blood vessels, and raises blood pressure; and (2) the parasympathetic nervous system that slows the heart rate, increases intestinal and gland activity, and relaxes sphincter muscles.

Symptoms associated with irregularity in the autonomic nervous system include unstable hypertension, excessively rapid heart rate, sweating, and pallor.

Azotemia. A higher than normal blood level of urea or other nitrogen-containing compounds in the blood. The hallmark test is the serum BUN (blood urea nitrogen) level. Usually caused by the inability of the kidney to excrete these compounds, azotemia is indicative of kidney failure.

Body mass index (BMI). A key index for relating body weight to height, the BMI is a person's weight in kilograms (kg) divided by their height in meters (m) squared.

The National Institutes of Health (NIH) now defines normal weight, overweight, and obesity according to the BMI rather than the traditional height/weight charts. Since the BMI describes the body weight relative to height, it correlates strongly (in adults) with the total body fat content.

Overweight Requires a BMI of 27.3% or more for women and 27.8% or more for men, according to the NIH.

Obesity Requires a BMI of 30 and above, according to the NIH. (A BMI of 30 is about 30 pounds overweight.)

Some very muscular people may have a high BMI without undue health risks.

Bradykinesia. Slowed ability to start and continue movements and impaired ability to adjust the body's position. A shuffling gait is one type of impaired movement. Bradykinesia is indicative of neurological disorders, particularly Parkinson's disease, or it may be a side effect of medications.

BUN. Blood urea nitrogen. A measure primarily of the urea level in blood. Urea is cleared by the kidney, and diseases that compromise the function of the kidney will frequently lead to increased blood levels. The blood BUN level can also rise in patients who are dehydrated.

Catabolism. Destructive metabolism; the breakdown of chemical compounds into more elementary principles by the body; an energy-producing metabolic process, the reverse of anabolism.

CNS (central nervous system). That part of the nervous system that consists of the brain and spinal cord. The central nervous system (CNS) is one of the two major divisions of the nervous system. The other is the peripheral nervous system (PNS), that part of the nervous system that lies outside the brain and spinal cord.

The peripheral nervous system (PNS) connects the central nervous system (CNS) to sensory organs (such as the eye and ear), other organs of the body, and to muscles, blood vessels, and glands. The peripheral nerves include the 12 cranial nerves, the spinal nerves and roots, and what are called the autonomic nerves that are concerned specifically with the regulation of the heart muscle, the muscles in blood vessel walls, and glands.

Creatinine clearance test. A test that helps determine whether the kidneys are functioning normally. Specifically, the creatinine-clearance test gauges the rate at which a waste, creatinine, is "cleared" from the blood by the kidneys. Creatinine is produced from the metabolism of protein as when muscles burn energy. Most creatinine is then filtered out of the blood by the kidneys and excreted in urine.

The rate of creatinine clearance is measured by first noting the volume of urine excreted in a given time period, such as 24 hours. Then the amount of creatinine in the excreted urine is measured and compared with the amount of creatinine circulating in the blood. If the kidneys are not removing enough creatinine, the level of creatinine in the urine will fall. Consequently, the level of creatinine in the blood will rise.

When the kidneys fail to clear enough creatinine and other wastes from the blood, the wastes build up in the bloodstream. Symptoms of kidney disease—including swelling (edema), nausea, and high blood pressure—may develop.

However, the creatinine-clearance test can usually detect waste buildup in the blood before it threatens the body. Doctors can then have an opportunity to eliminate the cause of the buildup and restore blood creatinine to normal levels. A creatinine-clearance test thus plays a key role in preventive medicine as well as in diagnostic and therapeutic medicine.

Calculating creatinine levels requires the following information:

A. The average volume in milliliters of urine excreted in one minute. (A milliliter is a metric unit equal to one-thousandth of a liter.)

B. The average amount of creatinine in milligrams in one liter of excreted urine. (A milligram is a metric unit equal to one-thousandth of a gram.)

C. The average amount of creatinine in milligrams in one deciliter of blood. (A deciliter is a metric unit equal to one-tenth of a liter.)

The creatinine-clearance rate is arrived at by first multiplying A by B, then dividing the result (product) by C.

The rate is expressed in milliliters per minute. Normal values for adult males range from about 110 to 120 milliliters per minute. Normal values for adult females range from about 100 to 110 milliliters per minute.

Decubitus ulcer. A bed sore, a skin ulcer, that comes from lying in one position too long so that the circulation in the skin is compromised by the pressure, particularly over a bony prominence such as the sacrum (sacral decubitus).

Delirium. A syndrome of impaired consciousness, attention, cognition, or perception. It develops acutely, often fluctuates over the course of the day, and is usually due to an underlying medical condition.

Dementia. A chronic, progressive illness characterized by loss of memory and a severe reduction in all aspects of mental functioning; significant loss of intellectual abilities such as memory capacity severe enough to interfere with social or occupational functioning.

Criteria for the diagnosis of dementia include impairment of attention, orientation, memory, judgment, language, motor and spatial skills, and function. By definition, dementia is not due to major depression or schizophrenia.

Dementia is reported in as many as one percent of adults 60 years of age. It has been estimated that the frequency of dementia doubles every five years after 60 years of age.

Alzheimer's disease is the most common cause of dementia. There are many other causes of dementia, including (in alphabetical order): AIDS (due to HIV infection), alcoholism (the dementia is due to thiamine deficiency), brain injury, brain tumors, Creutzfeldt-Jakob disease, dementia with Lewy bodies (tiny round structures made of proteins that develop within nerve cells in the brain), drug toxicity, encephalitis, meningitis, Pick disease (a slowly progressive deterioration of social skills and changes in personality leading to impairment of intellect, memory, and language), syphilis, thyroid disease (hypothyroidism), and vascular dementia (damage to the blood vessels leading to the brain).

Diaphoresia. Profuse sweating.

Diuretic. Anything that promotes the formation of urine by the kidney. The word "diuretic" comes from a combination of the Greek "dia" meaning thoroughly plus "ourein" meaning to urinate.

Diuresis may be due to a huge number of causes including metabolic conditions such as diabetes mellitus (in which the increased glucose level in the blood causes water to be lost in the urine), substances in food and drink (such as coffee, tea, and alcoholic beverages), and specific diuretic drugs.

All diuretic drugs (these are usually called, more simply, diuretics) cause a person to "lose water" but they do so by diverse means, including:

- Inhibiting the kidney's ability to reabsorb sodium, thus enhancing the loss of sodium in the urine. When sodium is lost in the urine, water goes with it. (This type of diuretic is called a high-ceiling diuretic or a loop diuretic.)
- Enhancing the excretion of both sodium and chloride in the urine so that water is excreted with them. This is how the thiazide diuretics work.
- Blocking the exchange of sodium for potassium, resulting in excretion of sodium and potassium but relatively little loss of potassium. These diuretics are therefore termed "potassium sparing diuretics."

Some diuretics work by still other mechanisms, and some diuretics have other effects and uses such as in treating hypertension.

The MedicineNet Pharmacy contains information on a number of diuretics including spironolatone (Aldactone), triamterene (Dyazide), hydrochlorothiazide (Hydrodiuril), furosemide (Lasix), and triamterene (Maxzide).

Dyskinesia. The presence of involuntary movements, such as the choreaform movements seen in some cases of rheumatic fever or the characteristic movements of tardive dyskinesia. Some forms of dyskinesia are a side effect of using certain medications, particularly L-Dopa and, in the case of tardive dyskinesia, the anti-psychotics.

Dysphagia. Difficulty in swallowing. Dysphagia is due to problems in nerve or muscle control. It is common, for example, after a stroke. Dysphagia compromises nutrition and hydration and may lead to aspiration pneumonia and dehydration.

Dystonia. Involuntary movements and prolonged muscle contraction resulting in twisting body motions, tremor, and abnormal posture. These movements may involve the entire body or only an isolated area. Symptoms may even be "task specific," such as writer's cramp. Dystonia can be inherited, can occur sporadically without any genetic pattern, or can be associated with medications or diseases (for example, a specific form of lung cancer). The gene responsible for at least one form of dystonia has recently been identified. Some types of dystonia respond to dopamine or can be controlled with sedative-type medications or surgery.

Edema. The swelling of soft tissues as a result of excess water accumulation.
Edema is often more prominent in the lower legs and feet toward the end of the day as a result of pooling of fluid from the upright position maintained during the day.

Electrolyte imbalance. A serious sodium and potassium imbalance that may cause cardiac arrest, kidney problems, or muscle spasms.
Oral electrolytes are a simple solution of water, minerals, salts, and carbohydrates. They balance the body's need for sodium, chloride, and potassium salts. These and other minerals change in the body into electrically charged particles called ions. If electrolytes are not perfectly balanced in the body, many organs, including the heart, cannot function properly. Electrolyte imbalances, if untreated, are fatal.
Electrolyte imbalance is often encountered in such conditions as heart failure, renal (kidney) disease, or cirrhosis of the liver and may also be aggravated by diuretics. Serum determinations of electrolytes should be performed and are particularly important if the patient is vomiting excessively or receiving fluids intravenously. Possible fluid and electrolyte imbalance may be indicated by such warning signs as dry mouth, thirst, weakness, lethargy, drowsiness, restlessness, muscle pain or cramps, muscular fatigue, hypotension, oliguria (less urination than normal), tachycardia, and gastrointestinal symptoms.

Encephalopathy (encephalopathic syndrome). A dangerous condition with s ymptoms similar to those of neuroleptic malignant syndrome (NMS), of which it may be a variant. It is associated with lithium toxicity.

Endocrinopathy. Literally, a disease of an endocrine gland. A medical term for a hormone problem. For example, hyperthyroidism, hypothyroidism, etc.

Extrapyramidal side effects (EPSs). These encompass a large group of clinical manifestations of overdose or individual sensitivity to a drug. They are believed to occur when there is excessive dopamine blockade in the basal ganglia. EPSs occur commonly in people being treated with long-acting neuroleptics. There are three main categories of EPSs: pseudoparkinsonism, dystonic reactions, and akathisia. Parkinsonism is characterized by motor stiffness, difficulty initiating movements, shuffling, stiff gait, resting tremors, and reduced facial movements. Dystonic reactions are acute, involuntary spasms of the muscles of the face (eyes, tongue) and back, manifesting as eye rolling, tongue protrusion, and opisthotonus. Akathisia is motor restlessness and manifests as pacing, rocking, and generalized agitation. Physical symptoms including tremor, slurred speech, akathesia, dystonia, anxiety, distress, paranoia, and bradyphrenia are primarily associated with improper dosing of or unusual reactions to neuroleptic (antipsychotic) medications. EPSs can be life-threatening.

Gastroenteritis. Inflammation of the stomach and the intestines. Can cause nausea and vomiting and/or diarrhea. Gastroenteritis has numerous causes including infectious organisms (viruses, bacteria, etc.), food poisoning, and stress.

Gastrointestinal reflux disease (GERD). The return of stomach contents back up into the esophagus. This frequently causes heartburn because of irritation of the esophagus by stomach acid. GERD can lead to scarring and stricture of the esophagus, requiring stretching (dilating) of the esophagus. 10% of patients with GERD develop Barrett's esophagus, which increases the risk of cancer of the esophagus. 80% of patients with GERD also have a hiatal hernia.

Glomular filtration rate. A measure of the kidney's ability to filter and to remove wastes or toxins.

Hematoma. An abnormal localized collection of blood in which the blood is usually clotted or partially clotted, usually situated within an organ or a soft tissue space, such as within a muscle.

A hematoma is caused by a break in the wall of a blood vessel. The break may be spontaneous, as in the case of an aneurysm, or caused by trauma.

The treatment depends on the location and size of the hematoma but involves draining the accumulated blood. A hematoma in or near the brain is particularly dangerous.

The word "hematoma" came into usage around 1850. It was devised from Greek roots: "hemat" referring to the blood plus "oma" meaning body; a bloody body or a collection of blood.

The many different kinds of hematomas are defined by location and include:

Epidural hematoma, a hematoma between the cranium (skull) and the brain's tissue-like covering, which is known as the "dura." Epidural hematoma is usually caused by a full-on blow to the head and is often associated with a skull fracture. Diagnosis is usually by CAT scan. Treatment is by trepanation: drilling through the skull to drain the excess blood.

Subdural hematoma, or bleeding into the subdural space between the brain and its tissue-like covering, the dura. If the hematoma causes increased pressure on the brain, slurred speech, impaired gait, and dizziness may result. Subdural hematomas can be caused by minor accidents to the head, by major trauma, or by spontaneous bursting of a blood vessel in the brain (aneurysm). They usually go unnoticed: when they do cause problems, the incident that caused the bleeding is often long past. Diagnosis is usually by CAT scan. Treatment is by trepanation: drilling through the skull to drain the excess blood.

Intracerebral hematoma, or bleeding and bruising within the brain. Diagnosis is usually by CAT scan. Treatment is by surgery.

Hypercalcemia. A higher-than-normal level of calcium in the blood. This can cause a number of nonspecific symptoms, including loss of appetite, nausea, thirst, fatigue, muscle weakness, restlessness, and confusion. Excessive intake of calcium may cause muscle weakness and constipation, affect the conduction of electrical impulses in the heart (heart block), lead to calcium stones (nephrocalcinosis) in the urinary tract, impair kidney function, and interfere with the absorption of iron, predisposing individuals to iron deficiency. According to the National Academy of Sciences, adequate intake of calcium is one gram daily for both men and women. The upper limit for calcium intake is 2.5 grams daily.

Hypercortisolism. Also known as Cushing's syndrome, this is a disease caused by increased production of cortisol, a hormone produced by the adrenal glands.

Hyperkalemia. Elevated blood potassium. Potassium is the major positive ion (cation) found inside cells. The chemical notation for potassium is K^+.

The proper level of potassium is essential for normal cell function. An abnormal increase (or decrease) of potassium can profoundly affect the nervous system and heart and, when extreme, can be fatal.

The normal blood potassium level is 3.5 - 5.0 milliEquivalents/liter (mEq/L), or in international units, 3.5 - 5.0 millimoles/liter (mmol/L).

Hypertension. High blood pressure, defined as a repeatedly elevated blood pressure exceeding 140 over 90 mmHg—a systolic pressure above 140 with a diastolic pressure above 90.

Chronic hypertension is a "silent" condition. Stealthy as a cat, it can cause blood vessel changes in the back of the eye (retina), abnormal thickening of the heart muscle, kidney failure, and brain damage.

For diagnosis, there is no substitute for measuring blood pressure. Not having your blood pressure checked (or checking it yourself) is an invitation to hypertension.

No specific cause for hypertension is found in 95% of cases.

Hypertension is treated with regular aerobic exercise, weight reduction (if overweight), salt restriction, and medications.

Hypertensive encephalopathy. An acute or subacute consequence of severe hypertension marked by headache, dulled perception, confusion, or stupor, with or without convulsions. Hypertensive encephalopathy is rare, given modern hypertensive treatment, and is a potentially rever-sible cerebral disorder occurring only in severe cases of hypertension.

Hyperthermia. 1) Overheating of the body due to extreme weather conditions. Unrelieved hyperthermia can lead to collapse and death, particularly in the elderly. Prevention via air conditioning, ventilation, and drinking extra water is the key for vulnerable persons. In emergency cases, injections of saline solution and rapid cooling of the body may be needed. Also known as heatstroke or heat prostration. 2) Medical treatment for cancer that involves heating a tumor or heating the whole body of the patient to kill cancerous cells.

Hyperthyroidism. Excess of thyroid hormone resulting from an overactive thyroid gland (or taking too much thyroid hormone). Symptoms can include increased heart rate, weight loss, depression, and cognitive slowing. Treatment is by medication, the use of radioactive iodine, thyroid surgery, or reducing the dose of thyroid hormone.

The thyroid gland is located in the front of the neck.

Hypertonia. Also known as spasticity. Increased tightness of muscle tone. Untreated hypertonia can lead to loss of function and deformity. Treatment is by physical and/or occupational therapy and in some cases muscle relaxant medication. Injections of botulism toxin (botox) are a recent treatment for chronic hypertonia in cerebral palsy and other disorders.

Hypoadrenalism. Also known as Addison's disease. Underactivity of the adenal glands. The adrenal glands are two small but very important glands, situated one above each kidney, which produce a range of hormones or "chemical messengers." Underactivity of the adrenal glands is called hypoadrenalism.

Many of the symptoms of hypoadrenalism are due to a deficiency of the steroid hormone cortisol, which is a potentially fatal deficiency if left uncorrected.

Hypocalcemia. Lower-than-normal blood calcium. Low blood calcium makes the nervous system highly irritable with tetany (spasms of the hands and feet, muscle cramps, abdominal cramps, overly active reflexes, etc.) Chronic calcium deficiency contributes to poor mineralization of bones, soft bones (osteomalacia), and osteoporosis, and in children, rickets and impaired growth. Food sources of calcium include dairy foods, some leafy green vegetables such as broccoli and collards, canned salmon, clams, oysters, calcium-fortified foods, and tofu. According to the National Academy of Sciences, adequate intake of calcium is one gram daily for both men and women. The upper limit for calcium intake is 2.5 grams daily.

Hypocortisolism. See "Hypoadrenalism."

Hypoglycemia. Low level of the sugar glucose in the blood, usually a complication of diabetes, in which the body does not produce enough insulin to fully metabolize glucose.

The symptoms of hypoglycemia include tiredness, dizziness, confusion, increased heart rate, and a cold, clammy feeling.

The treatment of hypoglycemia is careful diet, including eating small meals or snacks throughout the day, or changing the dose or timing of insulin or other drugs that affect blood sugar levels.

Hypothermia. Abnormally low body temperature. The condition needs treatment at body temperatures of 35C (95 F) or below and becomes life threatening below body temperatures of 32.2 C (90 F).

The signs and symptoms of hypothermia depend upon the body temperature. The major initial sign of hypothermia is a decrease in mental function that leads to impaired ability to make decisions. Tiredness or lethargy, changes in speech, and disorientation are typical. The person will act as if they are drunk.

The body gradually loses protective reflexes such as shivering, which is an important heat-generating defense. Other muscle functions also disappear so that the person cannot walk or stand. Eventually consciousness is lost.

Recognizing hypothermia can be difficult, for the symptoms at first resemble other causes of change in mental and motor functions such as diabetes, stroke, alcohol or drug use, etc. The most important thing is to think of the possibility and to be prepared to treat it.

Treatment involves slow heating of the body using blankets or other ways of increasing body warmth. Body temperature should increase by no more than a couple of degrees per hour. What is done for the hypothermic individual depends on the seriousness of the problem.

People with mild or moderate hypothermia who are alert and conscious and have not lost the shivering reflex will usually just require removal from the cold environment and providing additional insulation. The use of warm sleeping bags, lighting a fire, and warm foods and fluids are some of the various methods. Persons who have a more severe degree of body heat loss who aren't alert and can't shiver or stand should be brought to a medical facility as quickly as possible; rewarming of the body should continue as well.

Hypothermia is intentionally induced in some types of surgery and other situations in order to slow the metabolism of the patient and to decrease their need for oxygen during the procedure.

Hypothyroidism. Deficiency of thyroid hormone, which is normally made by the thyroid gland, located in the front of the neck:

Hypotonia. Decreased tone of skeletal muscles. In a word, floppiness. Hypotonia is a common finding in cerebral palsy and other neuromuscular disorders. Untreated hypotonia can lead to hip dislocation and other problems. Treatment is via physical therapy. In some cases braces may be needed to permit a full range of movement despite hypotonia.

Hypoxia. Concentration of oxygen in arterial blood that is less than normal. Anoxia refers to complete lack of oxygen.

Iatrogenic. The word "iatrogenic" comes from the Greek roots "iatros" meaning "the healer or physician" and "gennan" meaning "as a product of." An iatrogenic disease or condition is one that is inadvertently caused by a physician, a treatment, or a diagnostic procedure

Leukocytosis. Increase in the number of white blood cells.

Lumbar stenosis. A degenerative narrowing of the spinal canal, common in the elderly.

Meningitis. Inflammation of the meninges, usually due to a bacterial infection but sometimes from viral, protozoan, or other causes (in some cases the cause cannot be determined).

The onset is usually rapid (acute) and, if untreated, the disease can be fatal within a very short period of time. The early symptoms are non-specific and flu-like. They are followed by more serious symptoms, which may include rash, stiff neck, confusion, vomiting, loss of appetite, fever, headache, and coma.

Diagnosis is by observation of the clinical signs and symptoms and is confirmed by lumbar puncture to examine the cerebrospinal fluid.

Treatment depends on the cause of the inflammation. Meningitis can cause permanent damage to the brain and nervous system and is sometimes the cause of deafness.

Metabolic. Relating to metabolism, the whole range of biochemical processes that occur within us (or any living organism). Metabolism consists of anabolism (the buildup of substances) and catabolism (the breakdown of substances).

The term "metabolic" is often used to refer specifically to the breakdown of food and its transformation into energy.

Mitral valve prolapse. Drooping down or abnormal bulging of the mitral valve's cusps backward into the atrium during the contraction of the heart.

Myocardial infarction. The heart muscle (the myocardium) and the changes that occur in it due to sudden (acute) deprivation of circulating blood. The main change is death (necrosis) of myocardial tissue. An acute myocardial infarction (AMI) is a heart attack.

The interruption of blood is usually caused by arteriosclerosis with narrowing of the coronary arteries, the culminating event being a thrombosis (clot). The word "infarction" comes from the Latin "infarcire" meaning "to plug up or cram." It refers to the clogging of the artery. (The clogging frequently is initiated by cholesterol piling up on the inner wall of the blood vessels that distribute blood to the heart muscle.)

Neuroleptic malignant syndrome. The combination of catatonic rigidity, stupor, unstable blood pressure, fever, profuse sweating, and incontinence as a reaction to antipsychotic agents and therapeutic doses. NMS is a potentially fatal disease that occurs in 0.15% to 2.4% of patients receiving neuroleptic drugs.

NSAID. Non-steroidal anti-inflammatory medication, typically used for the inflammation of arthritis and other body tissues, such as in tendinitis and bursitis. Often implicated as the cause of adverse drug reactions.

Examples of NSAIDs include aspirin, indomethacin (Indocin), ibuprofen (Motrin), naproxen (Naprosyn), piroxicam (Feldene), and nabumetone (Relafen). The major side effects of NSAIDs are related to the gastrointestinal system. Some 10 to 50% of patients are unable to tolerate NSAID treatment because of side effects, including abdominal pain, diarrhea, bloating, heartburn, and upset stomach. Approximately 15% of patients on long-term NSAID treatment develop ulceration of the stomach and duodenum. Even though many of these patients with ulcers do not have symptoms and are unaware of their ulcers, they are at risk of developing serious ulcer complications such as bleeding or perforation of the stomach.

NSAIDs are taken regularly by approximately 33 million Americans!

The annual risk of serious complications is one to four percent with chronic NSAID treatment. The risk of complications is higher in elderly patients, in those with rheumatoid arthritis, in patients taking blood thinning medications (anticoagulants such as Coumadin and heparin) or prednisone (cortisone medication), and in patients with heart disease or a prior history of bleeding ulcers.

Oral rehydration therapy (ORT). A well-established therapy for treating dehydration resulting from vomiting and diarrhea. It involves replacing ongoing fluid losses from diarrhea and vomiting using an appropriate oral rehydration solution.

Oropharyngeal. Affecting the area of the throat at the back of the mouth.

Orthostatic hypotension. A temporary lowering of blood pressure (hypotension) due usually to suddenly standing up (orthostatic). Orthostatic hypotension, also called postural hypotension, may be experienced by healthy people (it is more common in older people) who rise quickly from a chair, especially after a meal. The change in position causes a temporary reduction in blood flow and therefore a shortage of oxygen to the brain. This leads to lightheadedness and, sometimes, a "black out" episode, a loss of consciousness.

Symptoms include dizziness, feeling about to black out, and tunnel vision (all due to insufficient blood flow to the brain). The symptoms are typically worse when standing and improve with lying down.

Tilt-table testing can be used to confirm orthostatic hypotension. Tilt-table testing involves placing the patient on a table with a foot-support. The table is tilted upward and blood pressure and pulse are measured while symptoms are recorded in various positions.

No treatment is needed for orthostatic hypotension. If someone with orthostatic hypotension faints, they will regain consciousness by simply sitting or lying down.

The person is thereafter advised to exercise caution and slow the process of changing positions from lying to sitting to standing. This simple technique can allow the body to adjust to the new position and permit the nerves of the legs to adjust to slower circulation in the older person.

Osmolality test, serum. Determines the balance between the water and the chemical substances dissolved in the blood.

Osteoporosis. Thinning of the bones with reduction in bone mass due to depletion of calcium and bone protein. Osteoporosis predisposes a person to fractures, which are often slow to heal and heal poorly. It is more common in older adults, particularly post-menopausal women, in patients on steroids, and in those who take steroidal drugs. Unchecked osteoporosis can lead to changes in posture, physical abnormality (particularly the form of hunched back known colloquially as "dowager's hump"), and decreased mobility.

Osteoporosis can be detected by using tests that measure bone density. Treatment of osteoporosis includes ensuring that the diet contains adequate calcium and other minerals needed to promote new bone growth and, for post-menopausal women, estrogen or combination hormone supplements.

Paresis (hyperactive reflexes). (1) Incomplete paralysis. (2) A form of neurosyphilis (syphilis affecting the central nervous system—the brain and spinal cord). Also known as general paresis, neurolues, acute syphilitic meningitis, meningovascular syphilis, tabes dorsalis, and the great pox. First recognized in Europe as a distinct epidemic in Naples in the late 1400s coincident with the invasion of Naples by the French. The dispersal of the debauched French mercenary army throughout Western Europe led to the frighteningly fast spread of the new disease.

Parkinsonism. An extra-pyramidal side effect caused by exposure to neuroleptic medications. Parkinsonism is characterized by motor stiffness, difficulty initiating movements, shuffling, stiff gait, resting tremors, and reduced facial movements.

Postural hypotension. See "Orthostatic hypotension."

Protein/energy malnutrition. A pathologic state characterized by inadequate intake of energy (calories) and protein; a deficiency of both protein and energy (i.e., calories).

Psychosis. A psychiatric illness or disorder. In the general sense, a mental illness that markedly interferes with a person's capacity to meet life's everyday demands. In a specific sense, it refers to a thought disorder in which reality testing is grossly impaired.

Symptoms can include seeing, hearing, smelling, or tasting things that are not there, paranoia, and delusional thoughts. Depending on the condition underlying the psychotic symptoms, symptoms may be constant or they may come and go. Psychosis can occur as a result of brain injury or disease and is seen particularly in schizophrenia and bipolar disorders. Psychotic symptoms can occur as a result of drug use, but this is not true psychosis. Diagnosis is by observation and interview.

Treatment is with neuroleptic medication, either the newer, safer, atypical neuroleptics like risperidone (brand name: Risperdal) or the older neuroleptics like haloperidol (brand name: Haldol.) In cases that do not respond to medication, electroshock therapy (ECT) is sometimes valuable.

Psychotropic drugs. Antipsychotics, along with antidepressants, antianxiety medications, and sedatives/hypnotics, belong to the larger category known as psychotropic drugs. These are the drugs most often implicated in adverse drug reactions, resulting in harm to the elderly.

Pulmonary embolism. The obstruction of the pulmonary artery or a branch of it leading to the lungs by a blood clot, usually from the leg, or foreign material causing sudden closure of the vessel. (Embolus is from the Greek "embolos" meaning "plug.")

The risk factors for pulmonary embolism include advanced age, cancer, genetic predisposition, immobilization (especially in the hospital), pelvic or leg trauma, pregnancy, and surgery.

The diagnosis of pulmonary embolism can be difficult because the symptoms are nonspecific and may mimic many other diseases. Pulmonary angiography is the gold standard test. Other tests may include oximetry and arterial blood gas analysis and imaging such as chest x-rays and ultrasonography.

The treatment includes anticoagulants such as heparin and warfarin (Coumadin). About 10 to 15% of patients with pulmonary embolism die.

Rhinitis. Irritation of the nose. Derived from the Greek word "rhinos" meaning "of the nose."

Sepsis. Also known as blood poisoning or septicemia. Commonly called a "bloodstream infection"; indicates the presence of bacteria (bacteremia) or other infectious organisms or their toxins in the blood (septicemia) or in other tissue of the body. Sepsis may be associated with clinical symptoms of systemic (bodywide) illness such as fever, chills, malaise (generally feeling "rotten"), low blood pressure, and mental status changes. Sepsis can be a serious situation, a life-threatening disease calling for urgent and comprehensive care. Treatment depends on the type of infection, but usually begins with antibiotics or similar medications.

Sinusitis. Inflammation of the lining membrane of any of the hollow areas (sinuses) of the bone of the skull around the nose. The sinuses are directly connected to the nasal cavities.

Syncope (fainting). Partial or complete loss of consciousness with interruption of awareness of oneself and one's surroundings. When the loss of consciousness is temporary and there is spontaneous recovery, it is referred to as "syncope" or, in nonmedical quarters, fainting. Syncope accounts for one in every 30 visits to an emergency room. It is pronounced "sin-ko-pea."

Syncope is due to a temporary reduction in blood flow and therefore a shortage of oxygen to the brain. This leads to lightheadedness or a "black out" episode, a loss of consciousness. Temporary impairment of the blood supply to the brain can be caused by heart conditions and by conditions that do not directly involve the heart:

Non-cardiac causes. Syncope is most commonly caused by conditions that do not directly involve the heart. These conditions include:

- Postural (orthostatic) hypotension. Drop in blood pressure due to changing body position to a more vertical position after lying or sitting
- Dehydration causing a decrease in blood volume
- Blood pressure medications leading to low blood pressure
- Diseases of the nerves in the legs of older people (especially with diabetes or Parkinson's disease) when poor tone of the nerves of the legs draws blood into the legs from the brain
- High altitude
- Brain stroke or "near-stroke" (transient ischemic attack)
- A migraine attack
- Fainting after certain situations (situational syncope) such as:
    - Blood drawing
    - Urinating (micturition syncope)
    - Defecating (defecation syncope)
    - Swallowing (swallowing syncope)
    - Coughing (cough syncope)

These situations trigger a reflex of the involuntary nervous system (the vasovagal reaction) that slows the heart and dilates blood vessels in the legs and causes one to feel nausea, sweating, or weakness just before fainting.

Cardiac causes. Heart conditions that can cause syncope or fainting due to temporary loss of consciousness include:

- Abnormal heart rhythms (heart beating too fast or too slow)
- Abnormalities of the heart valves (aortic stenosis or pulmonic valve stenosis)
- High blood pressure in the arteries supplying the lungs (pulmonary artery hypertension)
- Tears in the aorta (aortic dissection)
- Widespread disease of the heart muscle (cardiomyopathy)

To be sure, many of the causes of temporary loss of consciousness can be detected by a careful history. Dizziness after standing up in an older person suggests postural hypotension. Temporary loss of consciousness after urinating, defecaing, or coughing suggests situational syncope. Cardiac causes of temporary loss of consciousness such as aortic stenosis or cardiomyopathy are suggested by the occurrence of the event during exercise. Signs of weakness localized to certain areas of the body with temporary loss of consciousness suggest stroke.

Tachycardia. A rapid heart rate, usually defined as greater than 100 beats per minute. The tachycardias include sinus tachycardia, paroxymal atrial tachycardia (PAT), and ventricular tachycardia.

Sinus tachycardia is due to rapid firing of a normal structure called the sinoatrial (sinus) node, which is the natural pacemaker of the heart. Sinus tachycardia occurs in response to exercise, exertion, excitement, pain, fever, excessive thyroid hormone, low blood oxygen (hypoxia), stimulant drugs (such as caffeine and amphetamines), etc.

Paroxysmal atrial tachycardia (PAT) consists of bouts of rapid, regular heart beating originating in the atrium (upper chamber of the heart). This is often due to abnormalities in the AV node "relay station" that lead to rapid firing of electrical impulses from the atrium that bypass the AV node under certain conditions. These conditions include alcohol excess, stress, caffeine, overactive thyroid or excessive thyroid hormone intake, and certain drugs. PAT is an example of an arrhythmia where the abnormality is in the electrical system of the heart, while the heart muscle and valves may be normal.

Ventricular tachycardia is an abnormal heart rhythm that is rapid, regular, and originates from an area of the ventricle, the lower chamber of the heart. Ventricular tachycardias are most commonly associated with heart attacks or scarring of the heart muscle from previous heart attacks and are life threatening.

Tachypnea. An abnormally rapid (usually shallow) respiratory rate. The normal resting adult respiratory rate is 12-20 breaths/minute.

Tardive dyskinesia. A syndrome of potentially irreversible, involuntary, dyskinetic movements that may develop in patients who have been treated with antipsychotic medications longer-term. Some other drugs are known to cause tardive dyskinesia including tricyclic antidepressants, selegiline, clozapine, levamisole, and metoclopramide.

Xerostomia. Dry mouth. Xerostomia can be associated with systemic diseases (such as Sjogren's syndrome, systemic lupus erythematosus, rheumatoid arthritis, scleroderma, sarcoidosis, amyloidosis, hypothyroidism, and others). Xerostomia results from inadequate functionsed rather than constructions like "him or her." Indeed, since most family caregivers are themselves 60 or older, the information in this book will apply to their own healthcare as well.

Endnotes

CHAPTER ONE

1. Alliance for Aging Research, Medical Never-Never Land: 10 reasons why America is not ready for the coming age boom, 2002. Last accessed March 1, 2006 at www.agingresearch.org/advocacy/geriatrics/02016_aar_geriatrics_ text.pdf.

2. See the report at the link in the endnote above. According to this report, there are 76 million aging Baby Boomers in America today. Thirty years from now, those 65 years and older will represent one-fifth of the United States' population. The elderly account for a large share of the patient load of physicians. People 85 and older—the "old, old"—are the heaviest consumers of healthcare. They see a physician about 15 times a year, compared to about 11 visits for those over the age of 65, and 7 visits for those between 45 and 65.

As of right now, only 9,000 of the 650,000 licensed physicians practicing in the U.S.—fewer than two%—are certified in geriatrics. Worse, this number is shrinking as physicians retire or choose not to be re-certified. The problem is that Medicare payments fall woefully short as adequate compensation for the time it takes a doctor to assess and treat an elderly patient. Imagine—the usual elderly patient may have two, three, or more diseases or conditions. Medicare will pay a small amount for an appointment. That sum might be barely adequate compensation for a 10-minute visit. But most elderly patients should be seen for 45 minutes to an hour in order for a doctor to get a real handle on the changes in their condition and how their medications are or are not working for them. No wonder doctors are retiring from this field, and no wonder medical students aren't interested in pursuing geriatrics. There are other reasons why medical students can't and don't get trained in geriatrics. A major reason is that only three of the nation's 144 medical schools have a full department of geriatrics, and only 14 of these medical schools include geriatrics in their required courses.

While 86 medical schools offer an elective in geriatrics, only 3% of medical students choose to register for these courses. Let's face it: it's just not very appealing to consider treating the elderly patient. Many of them are sick or at death's door. Other areas of medicine are more satisfying and don't include getting involved on an intimate personal basis with a patient who's going to die fairly soon anyway.

The lack of doctors trained in geriatrics is only a small part of the problem. Only 720 of the nearly 200,000 pharmacists in the U.S. have geriatric certifications. This fact is shocking in light of the fact that the elderly are by far the largest users of pharmaceutical products. Fewer than 1% of registered nurses are certified in geriatrics, and less than 3% of advance care nurses specialize in the care of the elderly. Health providers in nursing homes—nurses, therapists such as physical and speech therapists, and aides—all lack training in geriatrics.

CHAPTER TWO

1. I have changed the name of the nursing home Mom was in for the simple reason that I don't want to be sued by the facility because it may disagree with my interpretation of its medical records and/or of conclusions I have reached in reliance upon studies and investigations in medical journals. For the same reason, I will use a generic term such as "antipsychotic" or the generic name of a drug rather than the brand name of drugs, except where several brand names of commonly used medications are given as examples.

2. Espino DV, Jules-Bradley AC, Johnston CL, Mouton CP. Diagnostic approach to the confused elderly patient. *Am Fam Physician.* 1998 Mar 15;57(6):1358–66. www.aafp.org/afp/980315ap/espino.html. When you see a statement like this that says, for example, "between 15 to 26%," it means that the statistics were derived from several studies. The lowest percent in any study was 15% and the highest percent in any study was 26%.

3. Tzepacz PT. Delirium. *Psychiatric Clinics of North America.* 1996;19(3): 429–448.

4. Id.

5. Espino DV, et al., supra.

6. Espino DV, et al., supra.

7. *Merck Manual*, section 6, chapter 76. www.merck.com/pubs/mmanual_home.

8. Espino DV, et al., supra; Jacobson S, Schreibman B. Behavioral and pharmacologic treatment of delirium. *Am Fam Physician.* 1997 Nov 15;56(8): 2005–2020. Lavizzo-Mourey R, Johnson J, and Stolley P. Risk factors for dehydration among elderly nursing home residents. *J Am Geriatr Soc.* 1988;36(2): 213–218.

9. Drug-induced delirium produces behavior that is often altered in different ways, depending on the drug. If sleeping pills are causing delirium, for example, the person may be withdrawn. Amphetamines, by contrast, may produce behaviors that are aggressive and/or hyperactive. Mom was taking several drugs that have delirium as a side effect.

10. Jacobson S, et al., supra; Bross MH, Tatum NO. Delirium in the elderly patient. *Am Fam Physician.* 1994 Nov 1; 50(6):1325–32.

11. Tueth MJ, Cheong JA. Delirium: Diagnosis and treatment in the older patient. *Geriatrics.* 1993;48(3):75–80; Jacobson S, et al., supra; Espino DV, et al., supra.

12. Espino DV, et al., supra.

13. Gurvich T, Cunningham JA. Appropriate use of psychotropic drugs in nursing homes. *Am Fam Physician.* 2000 Mar 1;61(5):437–46. www.aafp.org/afp/20000 301/1437.html; Kidder SW, supra; Siegler EL, Capezuti E, Maislin G, Baumgarten M, Evans L, Strumpf N. Effects of a restraint reduction intervention and OBRA '87 regulations on psychoactive drug use in nursing homes. *J Am Geriatr Soc.* 1997; 45:791–6.

14. Espino DV, et al., supra.

15. Dr. Mark Beers notes in the *Merck Manual* that an antipsychotic drug may be prescribed for a delirious patient who is aggressively paranoid or extremely fearful or to those who cannot be calmed with benzodiazepines such as Valium, but only as a means of resolving an acute problem on a short-term basis. Beers notes that antipsychotics must be used with extreme caution with elderly patients lest the drugs cause more agitation or confusion and/or mask an underlying problem. *Merck Manual,* Section 14, Chapter 171. www.merck.com/pubs/ manual/section14/chapter171/171b.htm Last accessed March 1, 2006.

16. Snader T. Appropriate use of antipsychotic agents in the treatment of behavioral symptoms of dementia. *HCFA Psychoactive Drugs.* Summer 1998, Vol. VI, No. 2. www.hcfa.gov/publications/newsletters/restraint/1998/rrspr98.htm. Last accessed March 1, 2006.

17. J. Consult Pharm, 1998 Feb; "Health Trends: Nursing Facility Top Ten Medications." There are no statistics available for later years. www.ascp.com/ public/pubs/tcp/1998/feb/healthtrends.shtml on Last accessed March 1, 2006.

18. Irizarry MC, Ghaemi SN, Lee-Cherry AR, Gomez-Isla T, Binetti G, Hyman BT, Growden JH. Risperidone treatment of behavioral disturbances in outpatients with dementia. *J Neuropsychiatry Clin Neurosci.* 1999 Summer;11(3): 336–342.

19. Id.

20. Tueth MJ, supra.

21. Espino DV, et al., supra.

22. Jacobson S, et al., supra.

CHAPTER THREE

1. Antipsychotics, along with antidepressants, antianxiety medications, and sedatives/hypnotics, belong to the larger category known as psychotropic drugs. These are the drugs most often implicated in adverse drug reactions, resulting in harm to the elderly. Gurwitz JH, Field TS, Avorn J, McCormick D, Jain S,

Eckler M, Benser M, Edmondson AC, Bates DW. Incidence and preventability of adverse drug events in nursing homes. *Am J Med.* 2000 Aug 1;109(2): 87–94. Often, as with Mom, nursing home residents and their families are completely unaware of the dangers these drugs pose.

In spite of this, psychotropic drugs, which have limited use in the elderly, maximum potency in the elderly, and are dangerous to the elderly, are frequently prescribed in nursing homes today.

Khan M, Farver D. Recognition, assessment and management of neuroleptic malignant syndrome. *S D J Med.* 2000 Sep;53(9):395–400; Scott BL. Evaluation and treatment of dystonia. *South Med J.* 2000 Aug;93(8):746-51.

2. Beers M., supra (1997); Gurvich T, et al., supra; Khan M, Farver D, supra; McDonough CM, Swift G, Managan B, Sheehan JD. Neuroleptic malignant syndrome: A diagnosis easily missed. *Ir Med J.* 2000 Jul–Aug;93(5):152–4. See also, Bajjoka I, Patel T, O'Sullivan T. Risperidone-induced neuroleptic malignant syndrome. *Ann Emerg Med.* 1997 Nov;30(5): 698–700; McDonough CM, Swift G, Managan B, Sheehan JD: Neuroleptic malignant syndrome: a diagnosis easily missed. *Ir Med J* 2000 Jul–Aug;93(5):152–4; Gleason PP, Conigliaro RL. Neuroleptic malignant syndrome with risperidone. *Pharmacotherapy.* 1997 May–Jun;17(3):617–21; Colón-Emeric C, White H. Case report: Catatonia and neuroleptic malignant syndrome in the nursing home. *Annals of Long-Term Care.* 1999;7(1):28–30; Bair BD. Presentation and recognition of common psychiatric disorders in the elderly. Clin Geriatr Med. 1994;10(2): 239–394. 2001 Aug. 9 (9).

3. Our request for withdrawal was not based upon any knowledge of the drug's dangers to Mom but rather on the belief that she was "not crazy" and that an antipsychotic was inappropriate. Here is a case where some education on the part of our family could have made a difference. It was only when Alpine Manor learned I would be transferring Mom to another facility that they finally—cold turkey—discontinued the medication.

4. Besdine RW, Beers MH, et al., supra; Gurwitz JH, Field TS, Avorn J, supra (2000).

5. The Institute for Safe Medication Practices (ISMP), a nonprofit organization, is dedicated to the safe use of medications through improvements in drug distribution, naming, packaging, labeling, and delivery system design. The ISMP works closely with healthcare practitioners and institutions, regulatory agencies, professional organizations, and the pharmaceutical industry to provide education about adverse drug events and their prevention. The Institute also partners with the FDA in MEDWATCH, an alert system for reporting of medication errors and adverse reactions, and regularly communicates with the FDA to help to prevent medication errors.

6. Besdine RW, Beers MH, et al., supra, citing Hepler CD, Strand LM. Opportunities and responsibilities in pharmaceutical care. *Am J Hosp Pharm.* 1990; 47:533–43.

7. Besdine RW, Beers MH, et al., supra.
8. Nananda C, Fanale JE, Kronholm P. The role of medication noncompliance and adverse drug reactions in hospitalizations of the elderly. *Arch Intern Med.* 1990;150(4):841–46.

CHAPTER FOUR

1. Holland EG, Degruy FV. Drug-induced disorders. *Am Fam Physician.* 1997 Nov 1;56(7):1781–8, 1791–2.
2. This definition is a combination of the definitions of the World Health Organization (WHO) and the American Society of Health-System Pharmacists (ASHP). "Requirements for adverse drug reaction reporting." Geneva: World Health Organization, 1975; American Society of Hospital Pharmacy. ASHP guidelines on adverse drug reaction monitoring and reporting. *Am J Health Syst Pharm.* 1995; 52:417–9.
3. Besdine RW, Beers MH, et al., supra; General Accounting Office (1996). Prescription drugs and the elderly: Many still receive potentially harmful drugs despite recent improvements. Washington, DC.
4. The "extrapyramidal" system refers to an area in the brain that is important in planning movements, but not in directly carrying them out, and includes the structures deep in the brain called "the basal ganglia." Problems with the extrapyramidal system are involved in movement disorders such as Parkinson's disease and Huntington's disease.
5. Irizarry MC, et al., supra.
6. Kidder, SW, supra.
7. Id.
8. Id.
9. Id.
10. Harris MJ, Panton D, Caligiuri MP, Krull AJ, Tran-Johnson TK, Jeste DV. High incidence of tardive dyskinesia in older outpatients on low doses of neuroleptics. *Psychopharmacol Bull.* 1992;28:87–92; Saltz BL, Kane JM, Woerner MG, Lieberman JA, Alvir JM, Blank K, Kahaner K, Foley C. Prospective study of tardive dyskinesia in the elderly. *Psychopharmacol Bull.* 1989;25:52–56.
11. Kidder SW, supra.
12. Id.
13. Casey DE. Tardive dyskinesia. In: Meltzer HY, ed. *Psychopharmacology: The Third Generation of Progress.* New York, NY: Raven; 1987:1411–1419; Jeste DV, Wyatt RJ. *Understanding and Treating Tardive Dyskinesia.* New York, NY: Guilford; 1982.
14. Holland EG, Degruy FV, supra.
15. Cooper JW. Adverse drug reaction-related hospitalizations of nursing facility patients: a four-year study. *South Med J.* 1999 May;92(5):485–90.

16. Id.
17. Forster AJ, Murff HJ, Peterson JF, Gandhi TK, Bates DW. The incidence and severity of adverse events affecting patients after discharge from the hospital. *Annals of Intern Med.* 2003 Feb 4;138(3):161–7.
18. Id.
19. Id.
20. Gurwitz JH, Field TS, Avorn J, et al. (2000).
21. Id.
22. Id.
23. The words "psychoactive" and "psychotropic" are used interchangeably
24. Gurwitz JH, Rochon P. (2002).
25. Gurwitz JH, Field TS, et al. (2003).
26. Dr. Mark H. Beers is the editor-in-chief of the *Merck Manual* and the *Merck Geriatric Manual* and a leader in the area of advocacy for the elderly, particularly as related to responsible medication use.
27. Beers MH, et al. (1991).
28. Beers M. (1997); Inappropriate prescribing for elderly Americans in a large outpatient populations, Curtis, Beers, et al., *Arch Intern Med.* 2004; 164:1621–1625.
29. Gurwitz, JH, Rochon, P. Improving the quality of medication use in elderly patients a not-so-simple prescription. *Arch Int Med.* 2002 August 12;162(15).
30. The URL for the website with package inserts for the top 200 prescription medications is www.mosbysdrugconsult.com/DrugConsult/Top_200/Drugs/e1916.html.

CHAPTER FIVE

1. Evans R. Trauma and falls. In: Sanders AB, ed. Emergency care of the elder person. St. Louis: Beverly Cracom Publications, 1996:153.
2. Siegler EL, Capezuti E, Maislin G, Baumgarten M, Evans L, Strumpf N. Effects of a restraint reduction intervention and OBRA '87 regulations on psychoactive drug use in nursing homes. *J Am Geriatr Soc.* 1997;45:791–6.
3. Kenzora JE, McCarthy RE, Lowell JD, Sledge CB. Hip fracture mortality: Relation to age, treatment, preoperative illness, time of surgery, and complications. *Clin Orthop.* 1984;186:45–56.
4. Thapa PB, Gideon P, Fought RL, Ray WA. Psychotropic drugs and risk of recurrent falls in ambulatory nursing home residents. *Am J Epidemiol.* 1995 Jul 15;142:202–11.
5. Id.
6. Id.
7. Steinweg KK. The changing approach to falls in the elderly. *Am Fam Physician.* 1997Nov 1;56(7):1815–1821.

8. Id.; Siegler EL, et al., supra.

9. Thapa PB, et al., supra.

10. Id.

11. The GOOGLE search "urinary incontinence" pads "home delivery" yielded 1,140 hits on March 1, 2006. (Contrast with 290 hits on Nov. 8, 2004.)

Chapter Six

1. Federal law requires nursing homes to make sure residents' hydration needs are met. Specifically:
   * Each resident must be assessed as to the adequacy of her nutrient and fluid intake.
   * Each resident must have a care plan, updated whenever there is a change in status, to address any specific nutritional or fluid deficiencies.
   * The nutritional and fluid status of each resident must be supervised by sufficient nursing staff.
   * The dietary needs of each resident are to be supervised by the resident's physician.
   * The resident must be provided with care and services required to maintain nutritional status. In other words, if necessary, assistance in eating and drinking must be given.
   * Each resident has the right to be free from physical and chemical restraints, which are known to decrease appetite and impede eating and fluid intake. Each resident is entitled to maintenance of her quality of life. This means facilities must ensure that each resident maintains "acceptable parameters of nutritional status, such as body weight and protein levels, unless the clinical condition demonstrates that this is not possible." Similarly, hydration must be maintained.
   * Residents with nutritional problems must be provided therapeutic diets. This is because a large portion of fluid intake occurs through food intake.

2. General Accounting Office 1996, supra.

3. Wick JY. Prevention and management of dehydration. *Consult Pharm.* 1999 Aug;14(8). www.ascp.com/public/pubs/tcp/1999/aug/prevention.shtml.

4. Burger and her associates have written a long article about their view of the "silent epidemic," focusing primarily on the dehydration, malnutrition, and significant understaffing perils endemic in U.S. nursing homes. Burger SJ, Kayser-Jones J, Prince J. Malnutrition and dehydration in nursing homes: Key issues in prevention and treatment. Commonwealth Fund. 2000 July; Pub No 386 www.nccnhr.org/pdf/burger_mal_386.pdf.

5. Lavizzo-Mourey R, et al., supra; Burger SJ, et al., supra (2000).

6. Wick JY, supra.

7. Id.

8. Kayser-Jones J, Schell E, Porter C, Paul S. Reliability of%age figures used to record the dietary intake of nursing home residents. *Nursing Home Medicine.* 1997;5(3):69–76.

9. Burger SJ, et al., supra (2000); Wick JY, supra.

10. Burger SJ, et al., supra (2000).

11. Id.; OBRA 1987 and OBRA 1990.

12. Burger SJ, et al., supra (2000); General Accounting Office 1996; Kidder SW, supra.

13. Electrolyte imbalance is an acute sodium and potassium imbalance that may cause cardiac arrest, kidney problems, or muscle spasms. Oral electrolytes are a simple solution of water, minerals, salts, and carbohydrates. They balance the body's need for sodium, chloride, and potassium salts. These and other minerals change in the body into electrically charged particles called ions.

14. I was able to use Mom's lab test results from her medical records and also the Internet calculator to determine her osmolality, which made it crystal clear that dehydration occurred, could and should have been detected by the staff at Alpine Manor, and most definitely should have been treated. I calculated Mom's osmolality at the beginning of her stay at Alpine Manor, finding that at 292, it was essentially normal. (Normal osmolality is 285 to 295.) Her osmolality calculated on October 10, about the time we noticed that Mom was again becoming delirious, was above normal (311), and the medical director noted in her records that Mom had an electrolyte imbalance. There was no evidence that this imbalance was treated. Another lab test was done on October 13 and the results (306) were still abnormal. But there was no lab work done to monitor her condition between October 13 and November 6, the day of her transfer.

On November 6, Alpine Manor again did lab tests, but inexplicably, they never gave them to me and they did not provide them to Mom's new doctor or nursing home. I obtained them many months after her death when I ordered copies of her medical records. Mom's osmolality on November 6 was 361, far above normal and a solid indicator of dehydration.

I also used the osmolality calculator on Mom's lab values for the date of November 13, when Mom was admitted to the hospital in multi-system failure. At 435 on that date, her osmolality was shocking. Later, on the Internet in a Continuing Medical Education segment for nurses, I found this statement:

> *Panic values for serum osmolality are values of less than 240 mOsm or greater than 321 mOsm. A serum of osmolality of 384 mOsm produces stupor. If the serum osmolality rises over 400 mOsm, the patient may have grand mal seizures.* **Values greater than 420 mOsm are fatal.** [My emphasis]

This material can be found on the Rnceus Interactive web site at www.rnceus.com/renal/renalosmo.html, Last accessed March 1, 2006.

15. The formula is:

    (2 x (Na + K)) + (BUN / 2.8) + (glucose / 18) for men.

    (2 x (Na + K)) + (BUN / 2.8) + (glucose / 18) X 85 for women.

16. Kamel HK, Thomas DR, Morley JE. Nutritional deficiencies in long-term care: Part II Management of protein energy malnutrition and dehydration. *Annals of Long-Term Care Online*. 1998 July;6(7):250.

17. Creatinine is a waste substance easily filtered by the kidneys and eliminated in the urine of healthy people. Kidneys filter creatinine from the blood at a given rate. Thus, the level of creatinine equals the glomerular filtration rate (GFR), or the rate at which the kidneys process blood through the glomerular system. If the kidneys are not working well, creatinine will accumulate in the blood. Thus, the level of creatinine in the blood as indicated in lab test values is an indicator of how well the kidneys are functioning.

18. Normal GFR is 85-125 mL/min. But, as we've discussed, there is a definite decrease in renal function as the body ages. According to Joel Shuster, PharmD., normal for Mom would have been "around 50–55 to 70–75 mL/min" [Email August 6, 2002].

19. Kamel HK, Thomas DR, Morley JE, supra.

CHAPTER SEVEN

1. Morley JE, Thomas DR, Kamel H, supra.

2. Burger SJ, et al., supra (2000).

3. Id.

4. Remember when you see a statement like this that it means it encompasses all studies from the ones finding the lowest percentage to those finding the highest percentage of malnourished residents.

5. Fiatarone MA, O'Neill EF, Ryan ND, Clements KM, Solares GR, Nelson ME, Roberts SB, Kehayias JJ, Lipsitz LA, Evans WJ. Exercise training and nutritional supplementation for physical frailty in very elderly people. *N Engl J Med*. 1994 Jun 23;330(25):1769–75; Burger SJ, et al., supra (2000).

6. Id.

7. Demling RH, DeSanti I, supra. Technically, this is called destructive metabolism, or catabolism.

8. Id.

9. Id.

10. Morley JE, Silver AJ, supra (1995).

11. Cole C, Bigando K, DeSutter S. Is altered nutritional status the root cause of your clients' negative outcomes? *J Nurs Care Qual*. 2000 Jan;14(2):41–56.

12. Gunning K, Saffel-Shrier S, Shane-McWhorter L. Medication use and nutritional status in elderly patients receiving home care. *Consult Pharm*. 1998; 8:897–911. www.ascp.com/public/pubs/tcp/1998/aug/rr.shtml.

13. The term "nutrients" is intended to include both food and fluids, as dehydration and malnutrition are interrelated.

14. Pinchofsky-Devin GD, Kaminski MV. Incidence of protein calorie malnutrition in the nursing home population. *J Am Coll of Nutr.* 1987 Apr;6(2): 109–112.

15. Burger SJ, et al., supra (2000).

16. Id.

17. Cole C, et al., supra; Demling RH, DeSanti L (a), supra.

18. Demling RH, DeSanti L (b). Protein-Energy Malnutrition, and the Nonhealing Cutaneous Wound. Nursing Clinical Management Vol. 3. www.medscape. com/Medscape/Nurses/ClinicalMgmt/CM.v03/public/index-CM.v03.html Last accessed March 1, 2006.

19. From the Level 1 Screen of the Nutrition Screening Initiative, a joint project of the American Academy of Family Physicians, the American Dietetic Association, and the National Council on Aging. Publications of the project include the *Nutrition Screening Manual for Professionals Caring for Older Americans.* The Nutrition Screening Initiative, 1010 Wisconsin Avenue NW, Suite 800, Washington DC 20007, (202) 625–1662.

20. Body mass index = Weight (kg)/(Height [in meters])^2. For example, someone who weighs 60 kg and is 160 cm tall has a body mass index of $(60/1.6^2) = 23$.

21. Demling RH, DeSanti L (b), supra.

22. Health Care Financing Administration, "Development and Validation of Measures and Indicators of Quality and Appropriateness of Services Rendered in Post Acute and Long-Term Care Settings: Statement of Work," 1998.

23. Health Care Financing Administration, "Evaluating the Use of Quality Indicators in the Long-Term Care Survey Process; Statement of Work."

24. Evans WJ. Aging and Malnutrition: Treatment guidelines. Nursing Clinical Management Vol 3. Accessed at Medscape http://www.medscape.com/Medscape/Nurses/ClinicalMgmt/CM.v03/public/index-CM.v03.html Last accessed March 1, 2006.

25. The conjunctiva is a membrane that lines the inside of the eyelids and extends over the front of the white part of the eye. It lubricates the eyeball.

26. Fiatarone MA, O'Neill EF, Ryan ND, Clements KM, Solares GR, Nelson ME, Roberts SB, Kehayias JJ, Lipsitz LA, Evans WJ. Exercise training and nutritional supplementation for physical frailty in very elderly people. *N Engl J Med.* 1994 Jun 23;330(25):1769–75.

27. Morley JE, Kraenzle D. Causes of weight loss in a community nursing home. *J Am Geriatr Soc.* 1994 Jun;42(6):583–5.

28. Kamel HK, Thomas DR, Morley JE, supra.

29. Kamel HK, Thomas DR, Morley JE, supra.

30. Rollins Carol J. Enteral nutrition, p. 202. Pharmacotherapy Self-Assessment Program. 4th Ed., American College of Clinical Pharmacy (2001) online at www.accp.com/p4b8samplemod2.pdf.

31. Id.
32. Id.

CHAPTER EIGHT

1. Report to Congress: Appropriateness of Minimum Nurse Staffing Ratios in Nursing Homes Phase II Final Report.
2. Institute of Medicine (IOM), Wunderlich GS, Kohler P, Eds. 2001. Improving the quality of long-term care. Washington, DC: National Academy of Sciences, IOM.
3. HCFA. Executive Report to Congress, 1998. "Appropriateness of minimum nurse staffing ratios in nursing homes."
4. Kayser-Jones J, Schell E, Porter C, supra (1997).
5. Harrington et al. 2000a
6. Kayser-Jones J, Schell, E, Porter C, Barbaraccia JC, Shaw H. Factors contributing to dehydration in nursing homes: Inadequate staffing and lack of professional supervision. *J Am Geriatr Soc.* 1999 Oct;47(10):1187–1194.
7. National Association of State Units on Aging. *Memo to the State Nutrition Contacts.* Washington, D.C., March 24, 1995.
8. Kayser-Jones J, Schell E, Porter C, supra (1999).
9. Id.
10. Id.
11. Department of Health and Human Services, Office of the Assistant Secretary for Planning and Evaluation, Administration on Aging. *Informal Caregiving: Compassion in Action* (June 1998). http://aspe.hhs.gov/daltcp/reports/carebro2.pdf Last accessed March 1, 2006.
12. Id.
13. IOM, 2001.
14. http://www.hcfa.gov/medicare. This Medicare website contains a free guide to choosing a nursing home, an interactive site where you can compare nursing homes in your area, a checklist for you to use when touring nursing homes, and information on alternatives to nursing home care. See also Appendix A available free of charge online at www.takingcharge-goodmedicalcarfortheelderly.com.
15. Nutrition Screening Initiative. *Screening Older American's Nutritional Health.* Washington, D.C. 1993.

CHAPTER NINE

1. A plebotomist is a specialist who deals with medical issues such as veinous punctures, insertions of IVs in troublesome veins, and so on.

2. Council on Scientific Affairs and Council on Ethical and Judicial Affairs. Persistent vegetative state and the decision to withdraw or withhold life support. JAMA. 1990;263:426–430; American College of Physicians Ethics Manual. 3rd ed. Ann Intern Med. 1992;117:947–960.

3. Nutrition and Hydration: Moral and Pastoral Reflections (Issued by the Committee for Pro-Life Activities of the National Conference of Catholic Bishops on April 1992) jmahoney.com/nutrition_and_hydration.htm#5.%20What%20role%20should%20.

4. Roig-Franzia, Manuel. "Catholic Stance on Tube-Feeding Is Evolving." Washington Post, March 27, 2005, final edition, via www.washington postcom.

5. Brophy v New Engl Sinai Hosp Inc, 398 Mass. 417, 497 N.E. 2d 626 (1986).

Epilogue

1. A Zone-aire ® is a special bed constructed with an air mattress with many baffles. It is used primarily for patients who are completely bed-ridden. The capacity to change the amount of air pressure in various sections of the bed is valuable for the purpose of preventing pressure sores.

Index

Index

About the Authors

JEANNE M. HANNAH, J.D.

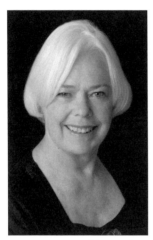 Jeanne M. Hannah graduated from the University of Michigan in 1963 with a B.A. in English Literature. She graduated Magna cum laude from the Detroit College of Law at the age of 45 in 1982. She is an attorney with 20 years experience as a lawyer. Ms. Hannah specializes in family law. Her research into the complex medical issues that pose life-threatening consequences for the frail elderly was prompted by her mother's death only 65 days after walking into a medical facility with a relatively minor urinary tract infection. The medical mismanagement, the devastating effects of medication errors, and the inexplicable failures to diagnose and treat what Ms. Hannah subsequently learned are common, treatable, and preventable diseases spawned a year of research and inspired this book to educate the armies of caregivers who are now or soon will be in the predicament faced by Ms. Hannah and her family and also to educate the millions of people over 50 who must learn now to avoid these common, life-threatening conditions.

While Ms. Hannah was initially intimidated by the complexities of the medical issues encountered with her mother, she has since learned that one does not require a medical degree in order to understand these common conditions that are prevalent and deadly to the elderly. She offers the reader encouragement, advice, hints for developing alliances with medical caregivers, and reassurance that medical problems in the elderly can best be resolved if caregivers are alert and use the tools provided in the book to help monitor their loved one's condition. Care recipients are empowered to speak out and to question the negative symptoms they are experiencing and the treatment they are receiving.

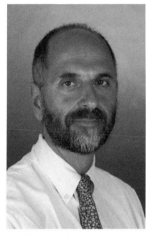

Dr. Joseph H. Friedman obtained his bachelor's degree at the University of Chicago in mathematics, master's degree in math from Washington University, MD from Columbia University College of Physicians and Surgeons, Neurology Residency at the Neurological Institute of New York, Columbia-Presbyterian Medical Center and then moved to Rhode Island in 1982.

Dr. Friedman is a Clinical Professor of Neurology in the Department of Clinical Neurosciences at Brown University Medical School. He is also the Director of NeuroHealth Parkinson's Disease and Movement Disorders Center in Warwick, Rhode Island. He is also the Editor in Chief of *Medicine and Health, Rhode Island* (the state medical journal, a joint publication of the Rhode Island Medical Society, Brown University, the Rhode Island Dept of Health and Rhode Island Quality Partners).

Dr. Friedman is also an elected member of the American Academy of Neurology Movement Disorders Section Executive Committee, and a fellow of the American Academy of Neurology Movement. In addition, Dr. Friedman is the clinical director of the American Parkinson Disease Association information and referral center in Rhode Island

Dr. Friedman pursues clinical research related to movement disorders, primarily Parkinson's disease, but also Huntington's disease, drug induced movement disorders, disease, etc. He has been involved in studying behavioral aspects of Parkinson's disease as his main focus. He is also interested in drug induced movement disorders, particularly those induced by antipsychotic drugs. He has been evaluating the atypical antipsychotic drugs in the treatment of drug induced psychosis in PD since 1984 and is involved, as PI of one multi center trial and as consultant in another. He has also been trying to better understand fatigue in PD, an area that has been little explored. Dr. Friedman and his colleagues collaborate extensively, and are currently involved in a study of a cholinesterase inhibiting drug to improve cognitive function in non-demented PD patients. They are participating in multicenter NIH funded studies evaluating the role of genetics in PD, and will be involved in clinical trials funded by the NIH of neuroprotective agents in PD, and in Huntington's disease.

A B O U T   T H E   T Y P E

The text of this book is set in
10.5/13.5 Goudy. The display is set in Goudy Bold,
Italic, and Small Caps,
with P22 Eagle Rock Extras ornaments
by Frank Lloyd Wright

C R E D I T S

Design and composition by Margaret M. Wagner
Photo of Jeanne M. Hannah by John Robert Williams
Photo of Dr. Joseph Friedman by Chuck Lusignan
Cover photo © 2006 JupiterImages Corporation

Printed by Thomson-Shore, Inc.
Dexter, Michigan